MW01247456

ADHD G⭐

ERIC ANDERSON

Dedication

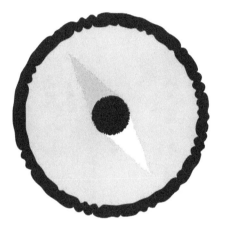

Dedicated to everyone who is struggling to see their own perfection.

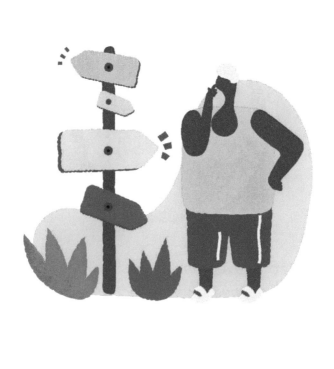

Contents

FOREWORD   11

ADHD BASICS   12

Introduction   13

1. Starting Out   15

2. Atypical   23

3. Main Symptoms   30

4. Causes & Impact   37

5. Diagnosis   43

6. Treatment Approach   50

ADHD TOOLS   62

Introduction   63

1. Principles & Critical Tools   65

2. Routines & Rituals   67

3. Calendar   70

4. Checklist   74

5. Notebook   76

6. Timer & Alarms   79

7. Launchpad   81

8. Visual Cues   83

9. Crossroad Moments 85

10. Rewards 87

ADHD BODY **90**

Introduction 91

1. Medication 93

2. Self-Medication 96

3. Environment 98

4. Sleep 103

5. Exercise 107

6. Diet 110

7. Meditation 114

8. Physiological Treatment Plan 117

ADHD BEHAVIOR **118**

Introduction 119

1. Reprogramming 120

2. Emotional Obstacles 123

3. Cognitive Obstacles 130

4. Behavioral Obstacles 135

5. Awareness 139

6. Thought & Emotion Record 144

7. Mantras 145

8. Remembering 147

9. Building Confidence 151

10. Motivation & Intention 153

11. Prioritizing 155

12. Goals 158

13. Planning 160

14. Progress 163

15. Play 164

16. Personal Style 166

17. Creativity 169

18. Behavioral Tactic Recap 172

19. Behavioral Treatment Plan 174

ADHD HOME **176**

Introduction 177

1. Responsibilities 178

2. Environment 180

3. Organization 182

4. Clutter 184

5. Losing Things 189

6. Chores 191

7. Finances 197

8. Time 199

9. Home Treatment Plan 201

ADHD SOCIAL **202**

Introduction 203

1. Communicating with Others 204

2. Friends 209

3. Significant Other 211

4. Social Treatment Plan 217

ADHD WORK & SCHOOL   **218**

Introduction   219

1. Obstacles   220

2. Coworkers, Clients & Workspace   225

3. Project Planning   226

4. Communication   229

5. Pay Attention   233

6. Follow Through   235

7. Finding the Right Path   237

8. Accommodations   240

9. School Tips   242

10. Workplace Tips   244

11. Work & School Action Plan   247

CONCLUSION   **248**

Awareness, Intention & Action   249

Foreword

Welcome to ADHD GO, a treatment program designed to help you overcome attention-related impairments and improve your life outcomes. With ADHD, your mind is in constant motion, but many of us also feel as if we're not getting anywhere; always going, but never arriving.

As people with ADHD, we need to approach challenges differently than others do. The first part of the book covers information about ADHD. The second part builds on that knowledge with specific treatments to help you adapt and navigate those challenges effectively.

Although this book is written for people with ADHD, the strategies presented are universally beneficial. Whether you are diagnosed with ADHD or simply want to modify problematic behaviors, the approach presented in this book can help.

ADHD GO is not a substitute for the help of a competent mental health professional, but it is an excellent starting point and a tool for change. Use the information provided as one element of your plan to improve your outlook, actions, and outcomes.

ADHD BASICS

Introduction

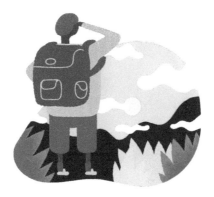

"Approach it and there is no beginning. Follow it and there is no end. You can't know it, but you can be it. At ease in your own life."

–Tao Te Ching, Lao Tzu

What most ADHD treatment misses is the work of overcoming years of subtle trauma that forced you to change yourself in order to fit into a system that wasn't built for your natural differences.

You don't need to change yourself. That's not the goal of treatment. You are perfect. Instead, you must change the distractions and self-delusions causing you to stray from your true self. Recognize that your problems result from behaviors that have accumulated over a lifetime; behaviors that were once useful defenses, but which now prevent you from moving forward and being at ease in your own life. Let go of the old fears and set yourself free. It's never too late and it's always the right moment.

The first step is understanding where you've been, where you are, and where you wish to go.

1. Starting Out

The problem

People with ADHD often feel wound up and struggle with certain skills. You might even feel like these "basic" skills are simply out of reach:

- Organizing and activating for tasks
- Sustaining and shifting focus
- Consciously regulating self-control

- Managing emotional responses
- Encoding and accessing learned information
- Monitoring and guiding your actions
- Managing time
- Attending to details
- Remembering things you were told

After years of floundering, the situation might seem hopeless, but these skills can be drastically improved with effective treatment. More importantly, you can escape the guilt and shame of the struggle.

The solution

You have a problem, but you are not the problem. The problem is a handful of maladaptive behaviors. You simply need to adapt your behaviors to fit the symptoms of your condition. You have not failed. You are not a failure.

- Pause, breathe, and accept.
- Deep inside, you know what must be done.
- Think about where you are going and why.
- Visualize your destination and connect with it on an emotional level.

Now, think of the bare minimum you could do to point yourself toward that destination. What's the smallest step you could take? Smaller. What's half of that? Half of the smallest possible step? If you want to read a book, don't sit down to read a whole chapter or even an entire page. Commit to reading just one word. Just think about taking a step. You're already doing it. Celebrate the small victories.

We are each heading toward different destinations but using the same tools and techniques to get there. Know your destination and learn the tools. What are you chasing? How will you proceed based on what you know about the road ahead?

My condition

Every boat leaks somewhere. Each leak is a symptom of the boat's overall condition. Your personal condition is defined by neurological symptoms. Experts have labeled a portion of those symptoms as ADHD (Attention Deficit Hyperactive Disorder). These symptoms last a lifetime and are on a spectrum of varying intensity. Fortunately, they are treatable and can even be beneficial in certain situations. You can't change yourself, but you can improve your condition and your outcomes.

Your condition is not defined exclusively by ADHD, but by everything that regularly influences your mental state: your emotions, thoughts, and actions. Recognize the ADHD as well as the other features that characterize your condition. What else is going on? Most people with ADHD deal with at least one other serious condition. These so-called "comorbidities" might include things like depression, anxiety, or bipolar disorder. Each must be treated separately.

No matter what the unique details of your condition are, this course will help you build resiliency, avoid setbacks, and move toward a life of greater personal fulfillment.

ADHD myths

Consider what you've heard about ADHD. What do you think about someone when you hear that they have ADHD?

Write it down:

When I learn someone has ADHD, I assume that they...

_____

_____

Myths about ADHD are more common than facts, so always get your information from a credible source. One common misconception is that ADHD isn't real. It is real. ADHD is caused by physical and neurochemical differences in the brain. Treating ADHD symptoms is as real and necessary as treating poor eyesight with glasses or asthma with an inhaler.

Another falsehood is that "everyone's a little bit ADHD." ADHD symptoms are an order of magnitude different in severity and duration from the normal inattentiveness experienced by the general population. ADHD symptoms consistently impair daily life and shouldn't be taken lightly.

Finally, some people claim that ADHD is a superpower. While the positive sentiment is welcome, ADHD comes with more challenges than inherent advantages. It's not a gift or a curse, but a condition that requires adaptation.

ADHD doesn't limit you or mean that you're dumb. It means you think differently. Many people with ADHD are highly intelligent, which often enables them to avoid diagnosis because they are able to hide their impairments.

The bottom line on ADHD myths is that you shouldn't listen to people who don't care about you and are not invested in your treatment. Everyone has an opinion that they will want to share for their own reasons. Shut that down. Only listen to yourself and your treatment team.

Here is a list of other common ADHD myths to watch out for:

- People with ADHD would be better off if they did things like everyone else.
- Anyone who really wants to learn should be able to sit still and pay attention.
- You should finish every project you start.
- You should start every project that grabs your interest.
- You should be responsible for doing all your own work.

- There are standard and inherently best ways to organize work.
- People with ADHD shouldn't be so sensitive.
- It's always best to reach your goal by the shortest route.
- People with ADHD are not as smart or capable.
- People with ADHD are deficient or disordered.

Don't allow misleading and bogus information to hurt your worldview. Be the gatekeeper in the garden of your mind. Below are some ADHD truths to keep in mind:

- ADHD is real.
- ADHD is not an excuse.
- ADHD is not a small, universal personality quirk like occasional forgetfulness.
- ADHD is not a gift or a curse.
- ADHD does not mean that you are dumb.
- ADHD does not limit your potential

Take it seriously

ADHD can be a life-threatening condition, especially when undiagnosed. People with ADHD suffer from higher rates of suicide, divorce, accidents, and joblessness. Don't write your symptoms off as quirks.

As with any treatment program, you get out what you put in. Your life can be 10% better tomorrow just by taking some small steps. You already know what to do; you just need to believe it will work for you. Go to the mirror, look yourself in the eye, and say, "I will not let you fail."

You are not alone

Currently, around 5% of the population are estimated to have ADHD. If you go into a room with twenty people in it, at least one of those people has ADHD, and probably many more. It is one of the most common neurodevelopmental conditions. Overdiagnosis has become a problem due to the influence of pharmaceutical companies, but no matter what numbers you choose to believe, the truth is that attention-related conditions are not unusual.

In any case, the purpose of this course is not to provide a diagnosis, but to help you manage problematic behaviors such as impulsivity, lack of consistency, and difficulty paying attention to details; things that people need to work on whether they have ADHD or not.

Atypical

Google defines neurotypical as "not displaying or characterized by autistic or other neurologically atypical patterns of thought or behavior." The accompanying example sentence reads, "neurotypical individuals often assume that their experience of the world is either the only one or the only correct one." This assumption causes a lot of problems for those of us who are not neurotypical, which includes people with ADHD. I refer to this group of people as *neuroatypical*, shortened to atypical for ease of use. Rather than refer to "people with ADHD or attention-related conditions," I will use the term, atypical, from here on out.

Unfortunately, atypicals also "often assume that their experience of the world is the only one," which causes us to dismiss chronic symptoms as normal. Instead of seeking help, we hide our problems, convinced that they stem from personal inadequacy. That is a sad, lonely, and false perspective.

Everyone has a condition. Yours is not only treatable but even comes with some benefits, so stay positive. Acceptance and compassion are fundamental to achieving successful outcomes.

2. Atypical

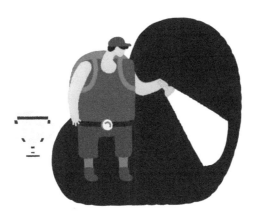

When I was growing up, a compassionate vocabulary for atypicals didn't exist; certain people were simply "special" or "different." Teachers referred to me as a "gifted underachiever."

I was naturally smart, witty, and outgoing, but my problematic characteristics were also undeniable. Hypersensitive, impulsive, distractible, disorganized, and constantly procrastinating. As a kid, those traits weren't deal breakers in most situations. In fact, they were kind of fun. I was outgoing and got into "fun trouble." I could bluff my way through tests and enjoyed shocking people into laughter with unfiltered outbursts.

As I got older, however, these characteristics no longer delighted people. Adult life is not a test you can bluff your way through. Things got serious and I could no longer rely on my wits without any preparation. I started to experience painful failures and harsh realities. Opportunities passed me by because people considered me unreliable, a wild card. I started to develop a sense of underachievement, which led to low self-esteem, guilt, and shame.

The longer these symptoms went untreated, the more problematic behaviors I developed to cope. Those behaviors led to more relationship problems and damage to my psyche.

I wanted to ignore it

Despite my mounting problems, I wanted to ignore their cause. It was easy to continue living as I always had, and, in the right circumstances, my impairments were advantageous. I was restless, but also curious. I was hyperactive but athletic. I was scattered but creative. I was impulsive and tactless, but also humorous and enthusiastic. Each negative had a positive interpretation.

Below are a few examples of traits that could have negative or positive interpretations:

- Restless/Curious
- Hyperactive/Athletic
- Scattered/Imaginative

- Fragile/Empathic
- Tactless/Outgoing
- Unorthodox/Creative
- Impulsive/Enthusiastic
- Forgetful/Easygoing

I didn't want to throw the good out with the bad. I identified with these traits as much as my eye color, my height, or my voice. They were parts of my identity that I didn't think could be changed even if I wanted to. This self-acceptance was largely positive, but it also prevented me from identifying ways that I could adapt and move through the world with less friction.

My symptoms snowballed in college. I was having trouble with relationships, skipping class, and neglecting my self-care. It was too much to handle on my own, prompting me to look for another way to handle the pressures of reality (besides binge drinking). I wanted a miracle cure.

Around that time, I started hearing about Adderall, a popular ADHD medication. Other students were referring to it as the "study drug." I thought, "That could be just what I need," and went to the campus clinic intending to get a prescription. To be clear: my purpose wasn't to get treatment for my condition, just to get a magic pill that would solve my problems.

The receptionist handed me an ADHD screening form, and I thought, "I'm just going to answer all of the questions in a way that makes them think I have ADHD," which turned out to be easier than I thought. Filling in the answers, I felt like anybody who took the screening would surely be diagnosed. I considered my life experience to be the norm, which prevented me from grasping the reality that my symptoms are not shared by everyone.

It is easy to unquestioningly assume that our personal experience is normal, whether that assumption is true or false. If you have never taken an ADHD screening, but suspect that you have ADHD, you might find yourself thinking, "Everybody deals with this stuff, right?" Wrong.

I was in denial about having ADHD but started taking the pills as recommended. For a while, it worked and I found myself doing a little better. My mind was clear. I started consistently going to class, doing my laundry, and getting things done without the mental fog or anxious paralysis I had grown accustomed to. It reminded me of squinting to see the blackboard, then being given glasses. I felt a surge of confidence and possibility.

Within a few weeks, however, I developed a tolerance for the medication. The initial euphoria receded and doubt crept in. Things returned to normal. I got depressed and started abusing my medication, chasing the lost magic of the pills.

Consequences piled up. Anxiety, guilt, depression, and shame obscured my positive qualities. Optimism was discarded in favor of tensing up for the next inevitable blow. I lived on constant alert. I loathed myself and blamed everything else. I lost my twinkle.

I had abandoned responsibility for my own treatment, becoming a powerless victim. I expected the medication to save me and overlooked a fundamental rule of treatment: Pills don't teach skills. That's the bottom line. Medication doesn't "cure" your condition. It gives you access to capabilities that are usually impaired by ADHD. It gives you leverage to do the hard work of changing old behaviors.

It's like learning to swim. The medication is like floaties around your arms. The little life jackets aren't going to be there forever, but while you're learning to swim, those floaties make the challenge feel manageable. You also need a swimming teacher; somebody who can throw a lifeline if they see you struggling. That's the basic idea of a treatment team. You are the most important part of that team because you are ultimately the one who needs to swim. Remember that learning to swim doesn't change who you are; it just gives you more options for moving through the world with ease.

Compassion changes perception

ADHD is a condition that carries plenty of shame, guilt, confusion and hardship. I couldn't ask for help. I didn't have the self-awareness, compassion, or the words to ask for what I needed.

I had accepted my suffering and was against seeking treatment. I was worried about the money, the time, and the stigma. I doubted the usefulness and was secretly embarrassed. I thought I could be my own therapist. After all, I'd gone to a professional before and nothing had changed.

Fortunately, my partner insisted that I talk to someone. She helped me look at options, get over my discomfort, and find the money and time. Her love and encouragement made it possible to seek the help I needed. We had unintentionally begun forming my treatment team.

I began to speak with therapists and a psychologist. I consciously surrounded myself with people who were positive about me and my condition. Not just positive, but excited. They focused on my potential more than my problems and taught me to do the same.

Challenge negative thoughts

Stop, breathe, and accept. Accept your circumstances and challenge the negative thoughts and emotions that assail you. They are illusions manufactured by your restless mind and will disappear under the light of level-headed scrutiny. Challenging your negative thoughts organically clears space for positive thoughts and emotions to take root and grow.

Remind yourself of your positive qualities. Some of those things will even be ADHD-related. Here's a list of some that may apply to you:

- Creativity
- Versatility
- Sense of humor
- Sharp focus
- Friendly
- Empathy
- Persuasiveness
- Zest for life

Your treatment team will help you enhance these qualities and use them to your advantage.

3. Main Symptoms

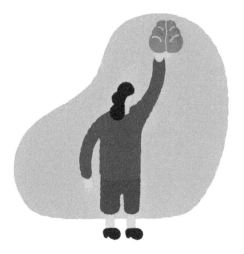

ADHD is a hereditary condition, which affects your thoughts, emotions, and behaviors. ADHD creates a state in which these internal processes are difficult to regulate consciously. You can't rely on your willpower or self-discipline to manage attention or emotional reactions, for example. These impairments typically manifest in unconscious operations and arise from differences in brain structure and neurochemical function.

I divide ADHD symptoms into three main categories:

- Contextual Attention
- Impaired Executive Function
- Hyperactivity

I'll also cover four sub-symptoms:

- Rejection Sensitive Dysphoria
- Oppositional Defiant Disorder
- Time Issues
- Memory Impairments

Finally, I'll end with a rundown of related issues, which arise from the main symptoms.

Contextual attention

ADHD is a condition of extremes. You're either on or off, particularly when it comes to your ability to focus. The quality of our attention depends on situational context, whether you're interested or not.

Under the right circumstances, you "hyperfocus" on a task. You don't go to the bathroom, you don't eat, and it's very difficult to switch tasks. You end up focusing on one thing at the expense of other important tasks.

The other side is zero focus. You're not able to activate your attention and you're bored. Your mind might be immobilized or scattered by little distractions. With zero focus, you're either paralyzed or working on so many things at once that you're not giving anything the attention it requires to be done well.

This symptom is most affected by external regulation. The pressure of an urgent deadline, for example, prompts some atypicals to flip from zero focus to hyperfocus. If you're writing a paper for school, you procrastinate until the day before it's due, then suddenly hyperfocus and finish just in time. Pounding the keyboard like a demon you might think, "This is just how I am. I do my best work under pressure." That might be true in some cases, but it's more likely an excuse for an unmanaged symptom.

Impaired executive function

You have an inner manager who handles a group of behaviors called executive functions, which include:

- *Activation* - Organizing, prioritizing and starting work
- *Focus* - Focusing, sustaining and shifting attention to tasks
- *Effort* - Regulating alertness, sustaining effort and speed
- *Emotion* - Managing frustration and other emotions

- *Memory* - Utilizing working memory and recalling information
- *Action* - Monitoring and self-regulating action

Unfortunately, your inner manager has a low tolerance for stress. Even small distractions can gradually sap your inner manager's ability to focus. When your inner manager is overwhelmed, everything becomes much more difficult. Suddenly, executive functions require twice as much effort. Cleaning your room goes from "challenging" to "impossible" in an instant.

Hyperactivity

Hyperactivity refers to a hyperactive mind, which puts our thoughts, actions, and physical sensations into hyperdrive. The combination of hyperactive thinking and low tolerance for stress often diminishes our reactions in high-stress situations to the most primitive options; fight, flight, or freeze. Your natural reaction is to blow up, shut down, or run away instead of thinking of the most appropriate response.

Physical and emotional sensations are over-prioritized in an atypical's mind. Light, sounds, smells as well as anger, sadness, or lust–any physical or emotional sensation–suddenly become top of mind and overwhelm everything else. We fixate on these stimuli and react impulsively because our internal manager is unavailable to help us regulate.

RSD & ODD

Two more conditions that stem from ADHD are worth mentioning here. The first is Rejection Sensitive Dysphoria (RSD), which describes an outsized reaction to feelings of rejection. The second is Oppositional Defiant Disorder (ODD), which is a reflexive intolerance of authority. You might not experience outsized reactions to rejection or authority, but it is very common.

Time issues

Atypicals live in the present moment. The future does not exist and the past fades as quickly as a dream. What's happening now is a hundred percent important and anything that's not happening now simply doesn't exist. There is only "now" and "not now." It's like having a tube up to your eye so you can only see what's right in front of you. You're walking and only looking at your feet.

Because the future doesn't seem to exist, it's difficult to set deadlines and accurately estimate when things will be done. We hyperfocus on the present moment because it feels as if each moment is infinite. Everything else can wait for the equally infinite "future moment," which may never arrive.

If time is like a river, then it is mostly whitewater rapids for atypicals. We feel it rushing around and through us, caught in a disorienting spin. Entire days disappear or stretch on endlessly. Part of the blame lies with insufficient planning, but it also reflects a fundamental difference in our relationship with time.

Memory impairment

Inattentiveness affects our ability to remember because we often don't focus on the details of an experience sufficiently to form a lasting memory in the first place. We rarely reflect on the details of past experiences because they are immediately being replaced by a new moment. The present moment is constantly arriving with new details, which are reflexively given priority. Deprioritizing the passing moment causes memories to rapidly fade into a general haze.

Insufficient working memory also causes us to pay insufficient attention to the emotions that we experience. Emotions shape our thoughts and future behaviors, which is especially important in regards to feelings of reward. A diminished experience of these feelings makes it difficult to learn from our experiences, recall relevant information, and plan for the future. We don't link memories to relevant emotional or practical information; therefore, we can't learn from our experiences without extra effort. We must focus on our memories and their associated emotions in order to retain them and learn from them.

These impairments are compounded by stress. Stress distracts us, making it even more likely that our memories and emotions will blend into one indistinct mass. Unconsciously discarding the nuance of our experiences, we are left with misleadingly simplistic memories that are tinted with a single, overarching emotion like anger, anxiety, or sadness.

Other issues related to the main symptoms:

- Difficulty with unwritten rules
- Talking louder than others
- The tendency to say what comes to mind without considering timing or appropriateness
- The tendency to worry needlessly and endlessly; a sense of insecurity
- Mood swings
- Inaccurate self-assessment
- Low self-esteem
- Inner restlessness
- Intolerance of boredom
- Frequent search for high stimulation
- Difficulty making and keeping friends
- Difficulty managing money
- Disliking traffic to the point of changing route
- Being fired from multiple jobs or changing jobs frequently
- Putting too many activities on the schedule
- Making a lot of lists but never using them
- Multiple speeding tickets
- Feelings of not living up to your potential
- See yourself as less powerful than others do
- Chronic procrastination
- Quick to get frustrated or angry

4. Causes & Impact

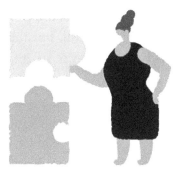

ADHD is a congenital, hereditary disorder caused by differences in brain structure and neurochemistry. Scientists continue to debate whether it is brain chemistry or brain structure that plays the dominant role.

Research about parts of the brain, their functions, and speculation on their relationship to ADHD symptoms is outside the scope of this book. This book is about treating the symptoms caused by these differences, not studying those differences for their own sake. Suffice it to say, your brain is different, but perfectly functional and doesn't have holes in it. Let's take a look at how these differences affect your ability to function.

Mental structure

A neurotypical mind is organized like a grid. Ideas, information, and emotions are all easily accessed and the connections are clear because related ideas are close together.

Atypicals, on the other hand, dump everything into one big pool, an idea soup where dissimilar ideas commingle and produce bizarre mutant offspring. This style of thinking has the potential to be inspired and useful, but the lack of structure means that locating specific pieces of information requires more time and effort.

Finally, because information is not coded by its relationship to other information, it lacks inherent prioritization; the hierarchy is flat. That means we tend to reflexively prioritize new information, making it impossible to ignore any stimuli because we unconsciously assume that it must be important.

Obstacles

Due to these neurological differences, atypicals are particularly susceptible to distraction from internal emotions and their external environment. Because emotional and environmental stimuli are difficult to ignore, they often cause problematic behaviors.

Internal distraction

Without awareness, our minds tend to fixate on emotions. We can unconsciously spend loads of time and energy manufacturing and analyzing unfounded thoughts which spring from unmanaged emotions, like shame, sadness, or anxiety.

External distraction

External distractions are sensory stimuli provided by your environment. Examples might be a barking dog, a strong smell, or a flickering light bulb.

Behavioral symptoms

Your reactions to internal and external distractions can lead to maladaptive symptoms like perfectionism, distractibility, and procrastination.

To overcome the problems caused by these obstacles, you need to deconstruct each behavioral pattern starting with the stimuli that triggers it. Observe the trigger, your reaction, and the result. We're often not consciously aware of our triggers because we've grown accustomed to them. Your reaction might be innocuous, but it can also be very destructive, especially when it serves no purpose. Consider how each pattern makes you feel. Ask, "How does it serve me?"

Impact

Your symptoms can affect all of your relationships: family, friends, co-workers, and your own self. Without awareness, you are at risk of gradually self-identifying as unreliable, inconsistent, unpredictable, even inconsiderate.

For example, you might blurt out thoughts or finish others' sentences because your own thoughts suddenly seem urgent and you worry they will be forgotten. However, that behavior is inconsiderate of the other person's thoughts and feelings.

When untreated, symptoms cause our relationships to become a source of anxiety which can cause us to retreat inward. We dismiss our good qualities and focus on the bad. When we don't feel good about ourselves, we can't relate to others. Sometimes it feels like the harder we try, the worse it gets, but you need to maintain a positive attitude because you can't heal in isolation. You must be able to be vulnerable with the people you trust, listen to their feedback, and appropriately express your needs.

Words to relearn

As we talk about obstacles, there are a few harmful words to eliminate from your vocabulary. Try substituting the harmful word with the replacement provided, so you can think positively about your condition.

Lazy → Insecure

Don't call yourself lazy or let other people put that label on you. It's not laziness that's stopping you from doing things; it's insecurity. You're afraid of the emotional outcome of authentically pursuing your desires, which causes you to avoid action. That's not laziness, it's self-preservation. Overcome your insecurity with curiosity.

Should → Feel obligated to

"Should" expresses an obligation, not a personal desire. It reflects external pressure from others. You will only actually do what you want to do. Remove "shoulds" from your life, or you will be paralyzed and miserable about the prospect of disappointing other people. Reduce the stress in your life and focus on "wants."

Stupid → Unfamiliar

Fear that you're not enough might cause you to choose the label of "stupid" instead. But you are not stupid and you are enough. You're just unfamiliar or unaware of how to get what you need. Again, replace your insecurity with curiosity. How can you get what you need?

Panic → Urgency

You don't need to panic just because something is urgent. Panic makes everything more difficult. It is a stressful, external pressure that arises from the fear of disappointing others. Urgency is internal and helps get things done on time. Working on tasks under last-minute pressure can cause us to associate urgency with panic, but panic is never helpful or necessary, even when working under pressure.

Failure → Not there yet

You haven't failed, you're just not there yet. Accept that it takes time to learn something and do it well. It's a natural process. The river must fill every bend in order. There are no shortcuts and there is no failure; there's only succeeding or giving up.

Drugs → Medication

ADHD medication is not drugs. It's medicine the same as an inhaler for an asthmatic, crutches for a broken leg, or glasses for vision impairment. It's not something to be sold to people who don't have prescriptions and are not under the guidance of a medical professional.

Disorder → Condition

Finally, you have a condition. I don't like that the last "D" of "ADHD" stands for disorder because it implies that atypicals are deficient. Your work and thoughts might be a little scattered, but that's a result of your condition, not because you are fundamentally broken or dysfunctional.

5. Diagnosis

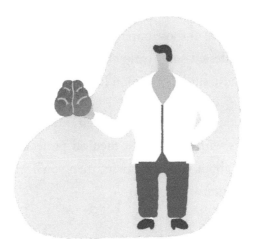

Getting an ADHD diagnosis is one of the most important steps on your treatment journey because it focuses your intention and begins the process of building your treatment team. It provides safe opportunities to practice discussing your condition.

Self-diagnosis is very simple and you can find a basic screening tool with a quick search online. Traditionally, there are two sets of questions to determine if you consistently exhibit inattentive and/or hyperactive behavior. If you score highly in either category, then you might have that subtype of ADHD.

You might also score highly on both, which could indicate the combined subtype.

Beyond simply exhibiting inattentive or hyperactive symptoms, you also need to have experienced them consistently since early childhood (age 7-12), and they must impair your life in more than one setting (home, school, work, social).

If you meet all three of those criteria (hyperactive or inattentive symptoms manifested since early childhood that impair your life) then you have sufficient reason to suspect ADHD.

You might decide self-diagnosis is enough and continue to treat your symptoms without seeing a medical professional, but if you are serious about your treatment, then you'll want to pursue a clinical diagnosis.

Clinical diagnosis

For most people with ADHD, it's difficult to research doctors, set appointments, get to the appointments, and deal with post-diagnosis feelings. Ask the doctor's office for a reminder call and recruit an ally to help with the other steps. Ask your significant other to help you set the appointment or even come with you. Bringing an ally can be very healing and provides a starting point for new conversations about treatment.

Allies can provide helpful background information to help reach an accurate diagnosis and provide emotional support.

Bring anything that can establish your medical history and behavior patterns such as current medications, past performance reports, or medical records.

One quick note on insurance: Using insurance creates a file in the Medical Insurance Bureau (MIB) database, which protects insurance companies from fraudulent claims. Pursuing an ADHD diagnosis may cause an insurance company to drop you because you are deemed too risky to cover. Because of this, some people choose to pay out of pocket, which ensures that no record is created. Check with your insurance provider before making your decision.

The diagnosis will take about an hour. Answer the clinician's questions honestly. They will, for example, ask about your drug and alcohol use. If you feel uncomfortable answering these questions, inform the clinician of your concern. Remember, this information is for the clinician to understand your circumstances, allowing them to make an accurate diagnosis and help you better.

Remember that getting a diagnosis doesn't "make you" anything. Don't be worried about being labeled forever; it is just information, an expert's analysis of what you're dealing with and what might help. You don't need to take their advice, but you do need to hear it.

Post-diagnosis feelings

After your diagnosis, you may experience a flood of emotions related to realizations about your life. You might cry, laugh, or become angry. Everyone's experience is different. Be aware that each step of the healing process takes time and energy. You may become exhausted during treatment from the emotional effort. This exhausted feeling is sometimes called a "therapy hangover."

You might find the stages of grief helpful in identifying emotions you may be feeling. Note that the stages do not represent stops on a linear progression.

- Denial → It's not true. The diagnosis is wrong. Everyone has ADHD.
- Anger → I should have known!
- Bargaining → God, remove this burden and I'll never sin again.
- Depression → I don't care about anything anymore.
- Acceptance → I have this. It's always been part of me. C'est la vie.

Regret and grief

You probably will feel regret for all the what-ifs. What if I had known earlier? You'll think of all the things you could have achieved, the relationships that wouldn't have broken apart, all the closed doors. But you'll get over that. You'll get stronger. The paths that are open to you now will become clearer, the obstacles easier to avoid, and the progress smoother.

Anger

You might feel anger that no one in your life identified your patterns of behavior sooner. Anger is a healthy emotion, intense and brief, like a cleansing fire. Unexpressed anger is dangerous when it becomes toxic resentment. Use your anger to speak hard truths and energize yourself for change.

It is important to forgive yourself and others. Everyone did the best they could at the time. When we know better, we do better.

Getting diagnosed allows you to view your behaviors from a more compassionate perspective. You have been dealing with a burden that you couldn't understand. There's been a stone in your shoe–or an extra weight in your backpack–preventing you from efficiently climbing your mountain.

Long-running patterns of behavior will suddenly be understood as obvious symptoms. A cluttered bedroom or piles of papers which were just "your quirky system" are now treatable behaviors, rather than a fundamental feature of your identity.

Whatever your emotional reaction, remember that it's valid and you don't need to justify your feelings to anyone. It's going to take time. Be compassionate with yourself. Make a conscious effort to be your own best friend during this time because you are meeting a new person who is about to form new relationships with everyone else in the world.

Answers people want

People are going to want answers to two fundamental questions:

1. "What caused this?"
The short answer is nature. It's hereditary.

2. "What does this mean for me?"
When you disclose your condition to your boss, significant other, friend, or coworker, you're essentially telling them that it may affect the relationship. You're asking for special understanding or accommodation from them and you need to be clear about what that entails. In most cases, it's not going to impact them whatsoever. Still, if you think that you're going to be asking that person for accommodations with certain things due to your condition from time to time, then you need to tell them the reason and reassure them that you'll be as clear and open with them as possible about your needs. That will improve the relationship because there are fewer unpleasant surprises.

Be very careful about those to whom you disclose your condition because, more often than not, disclosing your condition can become a personal liability. Only disclose to people that you trust or when it's absolutely necessary.

Learning how to answer these questions is going to help you feel safe and confident being yourself and will also help you learn to advocate for other people with behavioral conditions. You can help clear up the misconceptions that make life more difficult for all atypicals.

What's next?

Today is a new day. Not a fresh start. There are no fresh starts. But it's an opportunity to be free in a way that wasn't possible before.

Education

At this point, you might become hungry for information. Atypicals tend to like research because you can't fail at research. Hyperfocus causes us to become mini-experts on many subjects. Remember that knowledge is good, but action is better. Research is not action. Focus on developing new routines to treat your symptoms.

Action

You can encourage changes by rallying your family and friends. Start therapy or get coaching. Do not tolerate people who invalidate your diagnosis or the treatment, such as medication, which helps you deal with symptoms effectively.

Your relationships will change as you begin to manage the symptoms of your ADHD better.

The new me

You might reach a point when you are comfortable talking to people about your ADHD, a point when it is a natural part of your identity that doesn't define you. You are not just a person with ADHD. You are a mother, father, dancer, cool guy, whatever. It's yours to define.

6. Treatment Approach

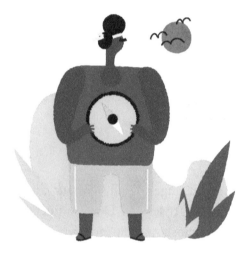

The ADHD GO treatment approach is self-coaching. Everything built by you and for you. It's got to be your plan because only your genuine emotional investment can sustain your forward momentum. A plan that you can execute and feel excited about every day for the rest of your life. You can have external account-ability all around you, but it's your effort and your daily actions–your choices–that are going to be the change.

Your ideal future self is not going to pop into existence from a momentary force of will, no matter how powerful. Your ideal future self is going to come from a commitment to years of routines that you enjoy avoiding. That's the grim reality. You don't manufacture a habit and set yourself on autopilot. You must choose to be your best self every moment. You must reach the point where you just are "the kind of person who always does X," where X is the sort of behavior that future you would do to become so cool. If your ideal future self has big muscles, then you just have to say, "I'm the kind of person who exercises every day."

Accept failure as part of the process. You will be beaten down regularly as you learn these lessons. You will often fail but never give up. Because of that, you will become resilient, and you will succeed.

Attitude

If you assign a number (based on its alphabetical order) to each letter in the word, "attitude," they add up to 100, which is a simple way to remember that your attitude determines everything.

Keep your thoughts positive and optimistic. Believe in the best possible future version of yourself, no matter how challenging or silly it might feel at times; you have nothing to lose but your despair. Even if people laugh at you, it's better than a future of inescapable regret.

Treatment team

"The biggest downside to ADHD for me is inertia. I know that I need to do something or change something, but many times I don't do it unless someone or something forces me to."

Your treatment team is the group of people who you can trust to be invested in your treatment outcomes. You are the most important part of your treatment team, but you can't do it alone. The following people are possible additions to your team:

- Best friend
- Significant other
- Therapist
- Coach
- Prescribing clinician
- Internet support groups

Each member of your team should be trusted to communicate honestly, hold you accountable, and encourage you. Their unbiased feedback might be harsh sometimes, but you must permit those people to be honest with you. Remember, you are fallible and will make mistakes; weakness is human. Ask for help and surround yourself with people who are excited about your potential.

The following are some characteristics:

- Listens

- Is knowledgeable

- Respects your rights

- Gives you recommendations and presents concerns

- You feel comfortable asking questions

- You can be honest and open

- You feel comfortable with the office environment and staff

- You feel comfortable bringing up alternative treatments

- Communicates in a reasonable amount of time

Don't listen to people who are negative or don't care about you and your treatment outcomes. Only listen to your treatment team.

Therapy and coaching

Therapy and coaching are both collaborative processes to help you move forward with your agenda; a creative process driven by you, and supported by the practitioner. Be honest with these professionals. If you aren't willing to fail, you will never succeed.

A therapist is different from a coach because they help untangle the emotional issues at the foundation of your unconscious behavior. They help to remove obstacles which lead you to self-sabotage. Talk therapies like CBT (cognitive behavioral therapy) and EMDR (eye movement desensitization and reprocessing) are both proven to be effective for overcoming trauma. Everyone has experienced some form of trauma, therefore it's nothing to be ashamed of. Treatment is a lifelong journey and a good therapist will be an indispensable ally.

A coach, on the other hand, focuses on the outcome of your actions, rather than the causes. They will hold you accountable, suggest tactics, and empower you to change. They listen to you, help discover your best courses of action, and provide additional accountability. They empower you to work on your plan.

Try several different practitioners until you find the right connection and allow some time to pass before judging your progress.

Structure and accountability

Structure and accountability are critical for establishing new routines. Structure gives you steps and screens distractions without relying on your willpower. Accountability gives you a reason and incentives for sticking with your plan.

Coaching contract

A contract is a set of criteria that you develop and agree to adhere to. It helps to have someone on your treatment team sign off on your contract for extra accountability. There are two parts of the contract:

1) Accountability plan

a) Send your coach a text after completing important tasks daily

b) Send a weekly email with success and stumbling blocks

c) Call the coach to update project status at least once a month

2) Rewards

- New toy
- Special coffee or food
- Event with friends to celebrate
- Sleeping in on the weekend

Your life is going to be broken down into goals and rewards that you will repeat for the rest of your life. That might sound boring, but it's actually liberating; it's simple, straightforward, and you get to choose the goals and rewards that you are excited about. How do you determine what you are excited about?

Treatment foundation

Transformative change relies on the emotions arising from your personal values. When we live our values, we experience feelings of reward, and those feelings are the fuel that motivates us to accomplish goals.

Humans are wired to alter their behavior around emotional responses. When we connect emotionally to our ideal future, it causes us to think and act differently.

Understanding the values that define your identity is the starting point. Start by writing down five. Examples could be family, freedom, creativity, financial security, or justice. With your values clearly articulated, you can begin to determine whether your life is in balance, and create a personalized treatment plan.

My values

1. _____

2. _____

3. _____

4. _____

5. _____

Balance

Balance is how we divide ourselves between different areas of our life. Balance is dynamic. Each area will have a different priority level and that will change. If your balance doesn't reflect your values, you're going to be stressed and unbalanced. Are you living in alignment with your values?

Rate your degree of satisfaction with each area of your life 1-10

- Career
- Money management
- Physical health
- Family and friends
- Significant other/romance
- Personal growth
- Fun and recreation
- Physical environment

Rating your satisfaction with each area of your life can help determine which areas require more attention. Working on one area often causes a ripple effect, which improves other areas too. For example, by focusing on your physical health, you may see an improvement in romance or recreation.

Goals

Your goals are the accomplishments that manifest your values. Write down a life goal based on each of your values. This list is not meant to be comprehensive, but it will solidify some of your abstract ideals. Once you have your goals written, visualize your future self after achieving those goals. Connect to that future self emotionally. Feel the pride of having attained those goals. Feel it so strongly that the feeling tugs you forward. Feel it pulling you, then turn your attention to removing any obstacles between you and that future reality.

My goals

1. _____

2. _____

3. _____

4. _____

5. _____

Treatment plan

When developing your treatment plan, address one symptom at a time. *Pareto's Principle* can help you choose which symptom to focus on first. *Pareto's Principle* states that 20% of your effort will yield 80% of the result. What symptom can you focus on that will have the biggest net effect?

Awareness of your target symptom is the first step of a successful treatment plan, which also includes your intention for change and the actions you take toward that change.

Awareness of the symptom you want to change

1. Example symptoms:

- Poor focus
- Poor switching
- Emotional dysregulation
- Impaired executive function
- Poor memory
- Poor sense of time
- Procrastination
- Perfectionism
- Fear of failure/success
- Inattentive, hyperactive, impulsive
- Context-dependent attention
- Positive illusory bias

2. Intention for a specific outcome

After choosing one symptom to focus on, decide how you want to reshape your associated behaviors. Get 10% better at managing the patterns around this symptom. Choose an emotional reason to improve and feel it deeply, helping you to remember the change when you feel like giving in to old habits.

3. Actions you take to reach the result

Challenge the symptom with action. Write down what happened, what you did, and how it went.

Aim for a 10% improvement. Don't expect 100% because you will fail and failure will hurt your ego and make you give up. You can't handle that yet. Build your cathedral brick by brick. Develop resilience with small, consistent victories. Try, then try something different. Find multiple ways to get what you need and don't give up.

Future vision

This whole plan is based on that vivid future vision of your ultimate self, your destiny. Imagine "future you" as a time-traveling mentor. What are they wearing? What's their job? Who do they hang out with? What's their day like? What did they accomplish that gives them that confident smile? Ask them. Feel their pride deep in your tummy. Make it your own pride. Feel it so strongly that you are drawn forward, attracted to that powerful sense of accomplishment.

Believe it, achieve it

Write it down, draw it, and speak it. That makes it real. The more energy and intention you put into something, the more likely that dream is to become real. Write down your values. Write down your goals. Write down your destiny. There will be obstacles along the way, and you will overcome them with curiosity and excitement. They are landmarks on your conquest of greatness. You cannot fail because you will not quit. Therefore, you must succeed.

Self-coaching vision

Based on your values and goals, write down details of the ideal future self that you envision. Begin to make your most hopeful vision a reality by writing it down.

Details about my ideal future self

_____

_____

_____

_____

_____

_____

ADHD TOOLS

Introduction

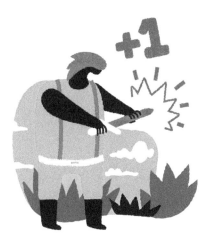

An important consideration which affects your treatment are the differences presented by your various life roles. Most people must play several different roles throughout the day, depending on responsibilities and social expectations. For example, our responsibilities could be very different depending on whether we are at work or at home. Likewise, the distractions you encounter, symptoms that arise, and treatments you have access to will also change. It's important to consider your different roles when doing things like making calendars or task lists. The following is a list of the most common roles.

How are things different when I'm at:

- *Home* - Homeowner, Spouse, Roommate, Parent, Child
- *Socially* - Friends, Acquaintances
- *Work & School* - Employee, Student, Boss, Teacher, Coworker, Coach
- *Alone* - Self-image

Treatments for each of these roles will be covered in subsequent chapters, but we'll start with critical treatment tools that are essential for your progress in any capacity.

1. Principles & Critical Tools

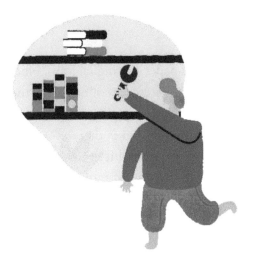

Critical treatment tools

Critical tools are the external reminders that are essential to strengthening your internal voice of accountability. You'll need these tools to establish the routines and resilience necessary to improve your life outcomes permanently:

- Rituals & Routines

- Calendar
- Checklist
- Notebook
- Timer & Alarms
- Visual Cues
- Launchpad
- Crossroads Moments
- Rewards

I use a combination of paper and digital tools. Find what works for you in that regard. External reminders are the key to following through consistently. Writing things down or speaking them aloud to other people makes them more real and creates an additional layer of accountability. A voice assistant like Siri, Alexa, or Bixby can help by making it easier to set reminders, timers, and make checklists.

None of these tools are going to make changes by themselves. They are simply structures that help screen distractions. You're not going to wake up tomorrow with new habits. New routines are easy to ignore, so it is OK to anticipate a struggle. It requires effort and conscious commitment to adapt your routines.

2. Routines & Rituals

Routines are a set sequence that you commit to doing, but which don't come naturally. A habit is something that it would feel strange *not* to do, like brushing your teeth. Habits are on automatic, while routines take effort. The truth is that the actions that will improve your life most might never be habits. Don't expect to reach a point where this isn't work. Stick with the difficult, but reliable reality of routines.

Rituals are routines that also elevate mundane actions of the sequence in some way. Rituals aid habit formation by imbuing your routines with more personal meaning, intention, and emotional power.

Exercise, work responsibilities, and household chores are examples of areas where rituals could help you remember your responsibilities with meaningful steps. How do you get into the right mindset to be intentional about how you spend your time? Consider all of your senses.

When approaching a routine, keep your daily cycle of energy in mind. What time of day do you typically have the right energy for this routine? Some people prefer to front-load their day with tasks they dislike most because they're sharpest and can push through more easily. That's called *eating your frogs for breakfast*.

Brain fog

Many people experience some "brain fog" in the afternoon, a period of mental fatigue after lunch. At that time, it can be beneficial to have other people around to help you stay focused. Schedule meetings, calls, and interactions in the afternoon, ensuring that you'll be less likely to space out.

Finally, when you do slow down during the day, use that time to regroup, review your progress, and recognize your accomplishments. That will give you more energy to move forward with clarity.

Check-ins

Your morning and evening routines are the most important rituals of all. These are the times you set aside to determine how you'll offer your energy to the world. Check-ins revolve around maintaining your calendar, notebook, and daily checklist.

At the morning check-in, transfer everything that is on your calendar and checklist for that day to paper. Doing so helps refresh your memory, ensures you're not overlooking anything and provides a convenient place to cross off completed items, which makes your progress obvious. Visualize the benefits of achieving what is on your list and the feelings of satisfaction that will come from being done.

At your evening check-in, review the day's accomplishments, reward yourself, and plan for tomorrow. Add anything to the calendar that may have popped up throughout the day. Determine tomorrow's goal and create tomorrow's task checklist. Finally, review your plan to make sure you haven't planned too much.

3. Calendar

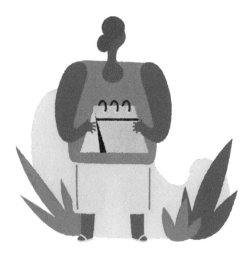

Calendars are a regular stumbling block for atypicals. It's difficult to set deadlines when your unconscious mind doesn't recognize that the future exists. It is our natural inclination to ignore the future during our moment-to-moment lives. That's why updating your calendar is so important. With practice, it will help you remain aware of the passage of time, visualize your destination, and respect your commitment to gradual daily progress.

Calendar structure

Start by putting deadlines for your main goals on the calendar, then work backward, setting regular milestones that are the necessary accomplishments on the way to reaching that goal.

This process is all about breaking your large projects into the smallest possible chunks and setting realistic timelines:

1. Choose a life goal–a destination–and set a deadline to achieve it.

2. Work backward to the present, breaking the goal into milestones, and milestones into actions.

3. Prioritize and estimate time to complete.

4. Move tomorrow's actions to your checklist.

5. Review, revise, and check time estimates.

6. Schedule transition time.

Goal-setting terms

- *Destination Deadline:* "By this date, I will achieve (life accomplishment)."

- *Monthly Milestones*: "By this date, I will achieve (monthly milestone), which moves me closer to achieving my destiny."

- *Weekly Accomplishments*: "This week, I will finish (accomplishment), which is necessary to achieve (milestone)."

- *Daily Tasks:* "Tomorrow, I will finish this check-list of tasks, which puts me on track to reaching my weekly accomplishment."

Write the steps required to complete each milestone on its calendar event, in order to remember what the project requires to be truly finished. Also consider the materials, obstacles, and help you might need. When will you prepare? When will you review the final details to ensure you haven't overlooked anything due to haste and carelessness?

Calendar tips

Keep separate calendars for each of your life roles or color-code your tasks by role to prevent any mixing of household chores with work or social obligations.

Plan fun first. We often neglect fun and relaxation when we're stressed. Fun is the reason we get up in the morning. It's the motivation for the work that we do and it is necessary to reach our goals. Put it on the calendar and plan your obligations around it and you will naturally focus on activities you are looking forward to.

Plan relaxation and transition time to reduce stress. Relaxation is different from fun, and it's important that you also have legitimate downtime. Transition times are short breaks between tasks. They can help ensure that you have time to switch focus so you'll be less likely to overbook yourself. We often overestimate what we can accomplish in a given time, which robs us of relaxation and causes stress.

Your calendar must be updated daily, so schedule time to schedule. Make it a part of your daily check-ins.

4. Checklist

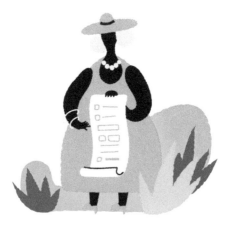

The daily checklist is a prioritized list of the tasks that you plan to finish today. These are the smallest possible chunks of work that are necessary to reaching your weekly accomplishment. Update your checklist every evening before bed. With your daily checklist ready for the coming day, you can go to sleep already prepared to spend your time effectively.

Consistently completing the actions on your daily checklist determines the velocity with which you are able to travel toward your life goals.

These tips will help you get the most out of your checklist:

- Date your list.
- Sort lists by role, just like your calendar (with colors).
- Prioritize tasks by their importance and their urgency.
- Estimate how long each task will take (nothing over 25 minutes).
- Keep a digital copy or small notepad that travels with you.
- If you foresee a time crunch, remove some items.
- Check off or highlight completed tasks and reward yourself.

Don't fall into an abusive relationship with your checklist. Keep it attainable by knowing your limits and not overwhelming yourself.

5. Notebook

Your notebook is the record of your progress and a place to clarify your thoughts. Keep your notebook visible, in the same place, and near a pen. You must be able to get to it quickly and record your thoughts to avoid any anxiety that you will forget something. Having a digital version can also be helpful, especially for quick notes when you are out of the house, but choose which one will be the master copy and be diligent about syncing the information to it.

Your notebook demands serious attention, so make it part of your morning and evening rituals. Schedule a meeting with yourself and take it as seriously as a meeting with another person. Set external reminders, like an alarm, to ensure you don't skip it.

Notebook structure

Organize your notebook into three main sections based on how often they are updated; annually, quarterly, and daily.

Section 1 - Annual

The broad strokes that define your trajectory for the coming year. Devote the first page of your notebook to the following entries.

- Values
- Future Vision Mission Statement
- Life Goals
- Positive Mantras

Section 2 - Quarterly

The quarterly section is a great place to expand monthly milestones into SMART goals:

- **Specific** - What exactly will you accomplish?
- **Measurable** - How will you know when it is accomplished?
- **Achievable** - Is it realistic that you can accomplish the goal based on available resources like time, skill, and materials?
- **Relevant** - Does accomplishing this goal advance my greater interests?
- **Time-based** - How long will this take?

Other entries could include evergreen items like grocery lists, household chores, passwords, car maintenance schedule, recipes, exercise routine, and any other static routines. You can keep this information in your quarterly or even annual section of your notebook.

- Milestone goals for this quarter (SMART)
- Lists
- Structures
- Rituals

Section 3 - Daily

The bulk of your notebook will be devoted to tear-out pages that you will use for updates about your wellbeing, current goal, and daily task list. You can also include "popcorn thoughts" that should be written down added to your calendar during check-in.

- This month's milestone goal
- Today's main goal
- Today's checklist → Digital checklist
- Popcorn thoughts

Finally, your notebook should be your resource for reflection and self-improvement. Below are some examples of other possible entries to include during your notebook time.

- Areas to improve
- Progress and setbacks
- Clarify thinking

6. Timer & Alarms

Timers and alarms help you stay on track and finish tasks on time. The passage of time is tricky for atypicals to pin down, so it's important to make it obvious. Timers and alarms are the most straightforward solution. Link your alarm to your current task by highlighting the task on your daily checklist or writing a sticky note placed near the timer.

Working in short sprints helps maintain focus through long projects because you can regroup after each sprint. More small victories. This method of short sprints and breaks is sometimes referred to as the *Pomodoro Technique*. Try working for 25-minute sessions with five-minute breaks at the end. Doing so will prevent you from getting burned out, which leads to frustration and giving up.

Analog clock

Clocks with hands make it easier to visualize how many minutes are left in the hour. That urgency is lost with digital clocks, which make the passage of time more abstract. Consider wearing an analog watch.

Bookend tasks

Bookend your tasks with an alarm set for the beginning of a task and the end of a task. Having a starting bell and an ending point reduces the overwhelming pressure of a long stretch of work. The breaks are warmups and warm downs to reward yourself, clear the last task away, open the new tasks materials, and consult your list.

Set limits

Your actions should be broken down small enough that none take more than a couple of short sprints (*Pomodoros*) to complete. Don't get frustrated if your estimates aren't accurate at first. This is an opportunity to learn what you can accomplish in a given period of time.

7. Launchpad

Your launchpad is your altar of important things; a place by the door for your keys, wallet, phone, lists, misplaced things, and small emergency items. If you consistently put your important things in one place, you will be less likely to misplace them.

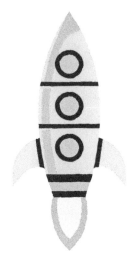

The launchpad is also a visual cue to pause for one final check before heading out. Stop, breathe, do a visual scan, and think about what you're about to go and do. This brief pause can help you remember to turn off the stove, grab your shopping list, or gather work materials that you might have forgotten.

Some possible items for your Launchpad include:

- Keys
- Wallet

- Phone
- Lists
- Flashlight
- Mask
- Water bottle

8. Visual Cues

Visual cues are stimuli that remind you of a behavior. For instance, if you always check the news when you see your phone, then the phone is a visual cue to check the news. It's a loop that you run unconsciously.

When you're aware of them, cues become powerful tools for creating new habits or preserving old ones. Consider all of your behaviors as patterns of triggers and loops. What stimuli are triggers for your behaviors? Learn to see the links, and you will be able to transition to more beneficial loops consciously.

Replacing old visual cues with new ones in your home or work environment can help you remember new behaviors. Display positive mantras, important lists, and calendars in prominent places. Make your reminders big and colorful. They should look fun. Dry erase markers are great for this too. You can write reminders on the car windshield, mirrors, and windows.

9. Crossroad Moments

Crossroad moments come right after a trigger, but before you follow a behavioral loop. For example, there is a moment right before you decide to surf social media instead of continuing your work when you think, "What the Hell, I'm going to indulge a little bit." That was the moment you stood at the crossroads. Learn to recognize those moments.

A crossroads moment could happen when you decide to hyper-focus on a task rather than eat, exercise, or sleep. This is the moment you need to watch out for, the moment you glance at the clock and justify putting off your self-care behavior for some shiny thing.

What patterns of behavior disrupt your self-care? What triggers did your environment provide? What crossroads moments precede those patterns? Look for recognizable signs of these moments.

Crossroads moments are the point when you start to feel as if you've seen this movie before. The familiar scenes where you allow your impulsivity to drive. Recognize the circumstances which accompany those strong enticements and manage your reaction to them. Ask yourself, "What's the benefit of the action I'm about to take?" Controlling your reactions is more difficult when we're feeling emotionally flooded, focusing on immediate gratification, or chasing something new.

If you can't avoid your triggers, try to delay your bad choice. Plan a short distraction like singing a little song or doing some push-ups. Shout a mantra like, "None shall pass!"

Writing down some facts about the situation can also help you make a more rational decision. Finally, don't punish yourself when you realize you've made the same familiar mistake; get back on track and commit to doing better next time.

10. Rewards

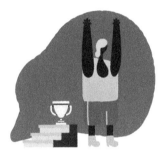

Negative reinforcement does not work. We can love ourselves and improve ourselves at the same time.

You should reward yourself for pursuing adaptive behaviors and achieving goals. Rewards emphasize positive behaviors and strengthen your internal self-regulation. Some people are more motivated by rewards and some are more motivated by consequences. Write a list of rewards and consequences that might work for you.

Rewards can be:

- Something you currently do and enjoy

- Things you would like to do or have
- Things you don't enjoy and would like to have taken away

Rewards that might work for me:

_____

_____

_____

Consequences can be:

- Something you currently do, but don't enjoy and could do more of
- Things you don't want to do but could benefit you
- Things you enjoy and wouldn't want to be taken away

Consequences that might work for me:

_____

_____

Use your distractions as rewards. For example, make mobile gaming a reward for a successful work session. Set limits on your "distraction rewards" and ask, "What am I rewarding myself for?"

Finally, make good behavior frictionless. For example, if you want to work out more often, keep the yoga mat or weights where they're visible and easy to pick up immediately. Conversely, you can add friction to behaviors you want to diminish. If you spend too much time playing mobile games, create a long password; anything that makes it slightly more difficult to pursue the distracting behavior.

ADHD BODY

Introduction

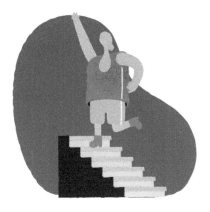

Your brain affects everything you do, and it is important to get excited about taking care of it. Physiological treatments enhance your natural abilities and reduce the detriments of your condition by altering your neurochemistry. Understanding your neurochemistry empowers you to consciously modulate it to improve treatment outcomes. For example, increasing dopamine levels can help increase focus and reduce anxiety, which drastically improves symptoms.

Common problems that impede physiological treatment are insufficient sleep, irregular nutrition, inconsistent exercise, overindulgence in strictly pleasurable distractions, and pursuing risky behaviors like drugs or dangerous thrills.

Your physiological state can also be affected by changes in the weather, temperature, seasons, life circumstances, screen time, stress, and recurring themes in your thoughts.

Physiological treatments are effective, simple to understand, and easy to implement. These treatments are also complementary, meaning you can do them all simultaneously for the best results. The more aware you become of how to modulate your neurochemistry, the greater your control of unconscious behaviors will become.

1. Medication

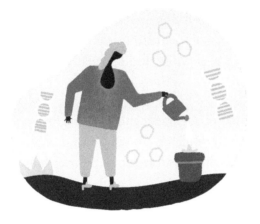

Your brain is physically and chemically different than a neurotypical brain. Just like someone with nearsightedness has physically different eyeballs and needs glasses, atypicals often require medication to normalize our functional ability.

Although different medications can be prescribed for specific aspects of your condition, the most common medications prescribed for ADHD are stimulants, which help correct a neurochemical imbalance. When used as advised, medication can remove obstacles that impair your ability to make meaningful life changes with few negative side-effects.

There are many types of medication and each will have different effects on different people, which means it's important to work with a trained professional and be open to trying several options until you find what's right for you.

Take your medication regularly and monitor the effects. Most people who start a medication will have an initial period of euphoria, followed by a gradual acclimation to the medication. This is normal and means that the medication is working as intended. You're still benefiting from the medication's effects even without the euphoric feelings that you might experience initially.

Remember that taking medication is not a lifelong, permanent decision. Most stimulants are safe to quit at any time. These medications are intended as support for as long as you need them, similar to crutches during the early stages of physical therapy. Ideally, you can take medication as you develop stronger habits and then stop. It's also common to take "medication vacations," which are times when you are experiencing low stress and can manage your symptoms without medication.

Finally, *everything* is expensive, has some side effects, and is insufficient–by itself–to change your life for the better. These are imperfect tools, but can be hugely beneficial when used with understanding and intention.

Concerns

Many people have ideological concerns about taking medication. Some of the most common concerns can be alleviated by understanding what you take and why you're taking it. We use any tool intending to facilitate positive outcomes.

Understand the trade-offs and watch for common side effects.

Also, don't abuse your medication or sell it. This creates personal problems, adds to negative misconceptions about ADHD, and leads to tighter restrictions on vital medicines.

Remember to take it

Take your medication exactly as prescribed and on time. Set an alarm to remember to take your meds on schedule. Remember that you took it by fixing the memory of taking it in your mind or using a med caddy. Take them with you. Keep up on refills.

Pills don't teach skills

The purpose of medication is to facilitate more adaptive behaviors. The medication will not do the work of changing your behaviors by magic. Know what you take and understand exactly how it can help you tackle specific symptoms.

2. Self-Medication

What gives you a rush or puts you in a state of flow? That's medicine.

Understanding the options available to regulate your brain chemistry responsibly and without prescription drugs can be a vital part of treatment. Our brains naturally release dopamine during emotionally or physically intense experiences. Examples could include sex, dancing, engaging in stimulating conversation, or just watching an emotional movie.

Atypicals also turn to drugs like cannabis, nicotine, and alcohol to artificially alter their brain chemistry. Unfortunately, this method of self-medication contributes to notably higher levels of addiction among atypicals. Studies have shown that substance abuse is more common when ADHD is untreated, which suggests that medication can provide a positive alternative.

As with prescription medication, practice intention and awareness. Know what you are using and why. Don't become addicted to mindless escapism like porn, games, and drugs. Consider the consequences.

The golden rule of self-medication is: don't put yourself (or others) in danger and don't overdo it.

3. Environment

An environment is a collection of stimuli that shape our experience and behaviors. The patterns that define our lives begin with the stimuli provided by our environments. With that in mind, choosing the right environment can be the most consequential decision you make.

The ideal environment is somewhere you feel secure, comfortable, and able to limit distractions. It is helpful to have a specific environment for each of your roles or types of tasks; where you relax should not be where you work, for example. Your environment should also provide access to resources that can help with things you are not good at, like people who inspire you and hold you accountable. Consider whether you want to be solely responsible for holding yourself accountable. This can be a dangerous amount of freedom.

Prepare the space by organizing the materials you need for your current task and keeping all other visual clutter out of sight. Visual clutter saps focus energy and increases the likelihood of distraction. In addition to a clean workplace, make sure your bag and materials are clean and well organized. Be aware of your "clutter decisions," moments when you avoid putting something in its proper place and add to the clutter, and strive to make more anti-clutter decisions.

Accept that distractions are impossible to eliminate entirely, but take control where you can. For example, bring snacks and drinks to limit the number of times you need to get up. Also, set limits for the time you will allow for electronic distractions like checking your phone.

Evaluate your current environment for distractions and consider each of your senses:

Sight (lighting, decorations)

_____

_____

Sound (white noise, music, random sounds)

_____

_____

Smell

_____

_____

Feel (temperature, humidity, furniture)

_____

_____

Many distractions we unconsciously ignore, but they still cause problems. Which is most distracting for you in particular: loud noises or a blinking light? The smell of food or a chair that is too tall?

Now visualize your ideal environment. How is it different from your current environment? What is the ideal environment for the task you need to perform?

Environment planning

Take all of your senses into consideration. *Feng Shui* can be a fun set of principles to organize your environment around because it provides structure. Here are some examples of environmental considerations:

Walls

- Art - Serene art on the walls and soothing wall colors, inspirational mantras
- Furnishings - Soft cushions, rocking or swinging chair, big cushion or memory foam pad with a cover, small piece of carpet or rug, aquarium, indoor plants

- Lighting - Rock-salt lamps, candles, warm light
- Climate - Comfortable temperature and humidity

Soundscape

- Noise-canceling headphones
- Soothing music playlists
- Instrumental
- Uptempo and downtempo
- Binaural
- Nature sounds
- Chimes
- Water fountain
- Fans
- White-noise machines

Smells

- Aromatherapy candles or incense
- Essential oils
- Fresh air from the window

Snacks

Snacking can help you focus, but make sure you plan what you'll snack on or you can stack up calories quickly.

- Snack basket
- Tea station with electric kettle

Intentional distractions

- Basket of fidgets (like knitting) to play with
- A pet or stuffed animal to cheer you
- Exercise mat or weights

Organizational systems

Keep things out of sight when they are not in use to prevent them from becoming distractions.

4. Sleep

Good sleep hygiene increases attention, reduces irritability, improves memory, reduces stress, contributes to quicker thinking, and facilitates the acquisition of new information. Most people need eight hours to get the maximum brain-boosting benefit from sleep.

Sleeping and waking at the same time every day is also important for establishing your circadian rhythm because it keeps your level of alertness consistent and predictable. Beyond simply determining whether you are a night owl or morning person, look for patterns throughout your day. For example, most people are sharpest in the morning, then get a little foggy for a few hours after lunch.

The night owl fallacy

Bored all day then, just before bed, everything is interesting. Bored and tired most of the time.

Many atypicals believe they are night owls. We can spend the whole day feeling unable to accomplish an important task, but, when the workday is over, stay up all night doing a range of activities with vigor.

The paralysis we experience during the day arises from our pre-occupation with what we "should" be doing. After the sun goes down and our workday responsibilities fade, however, we are free to do the things we actually wanted to be doing all day. When our "shoulds" are deprioritized, all of that pressure is cleared away, making room for curiosity and real attention.

Don't fall into the trap of letting "shoulds" keep you in a sleep-deprived cycle. Replace "shoulds" with "wants" in your day. Being more authentic with your desires during the day will allow you to do things you care about when you are more alert, and you will get the benefits of more consistent sleep.

Getting to sleep

Make your bedroom a designated sleep room. It should be comfy and you should have access to sleep aids like earplugs, white noise, blackout curtains, and be kept at an ideal temperature for you. Other sleep aids include:

- Boring books
- Warm bath
- Backrub
- Soft music or nature sounds

- Restrictive bedding like a weighted blanket
- Warm milk
- Hypnosis
- Light snack

Create a bedtime routine and keep a consistent bedtime. Set a bedtime alarm to start getting ready for bed early.

One of the biggest obstacles to sleep these days is treating our bedrooms like movie theatres. Don't spend time in your bedroom if you do not intend to be asleep. Move electronics out of there. Other sleep distractions include:

- TV before bed
- Active play
- A big meal before bed
- Exercise late in the day
- Drugs before bed
- Naps before bed
- Medication-related issues

If you can't fall asleep, don't lie awake for hours in bed. Get up but stay relaxed and avoid screens.

Waking up

Waking up should be its own ritual. Here are some suggestions to help you start the day with enthusiasm:

- Set your alarm to play music.

- Keep the alarm out of the room.

- Take your meds before you're supposed to get out of bed.

- Don't lie awake for hours in bed, it's a common anxiety trap.

- Get up, but keep it relaxing and ease into the day.

- Start the day with something that motivates you.

- Stay away from early classes and other obligations.

- Your demons hate fresh air and sunlight, take a walk.

5. Exercise

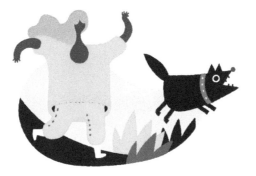

Your body is a reflection of your unconscious thoughts and habits. Taking care of your body reflects good habits and self-esteem.

Even if you're not interested in feeling good and looking good, exercise is proven to boost your focus for a few hours afterward. Just 30 to 60 minutes of repetitive motion each day. Remember that you can break it into chunks and that the little things you build into your daily routine will make a big difference. Take the stairs instead of the elevator, for instance.

Ease into it and choose something that is at your ability level. Set a reasonable minimum and maximum goal for yourself. Be intentional about how you use the time. It's helpful to get a partner or a trainer to hold you accountable because the hardest part of exercising is simply getting started each day.

For some people, consistency is key. Some people prefer to break it up and have spontaneous "mini-workouts" throughout their day. Keep it flexible if that works for you. Anything is better than nothing. Whether you're consistent or flexible, don't tolerate any excuse to do nothing.

Exercise suggestions

- Calf-raises
- Heel touches
- Lunges
- Triceps dips
- Push-ups
- Sit-ups
- Squats
- Chin-ups
- Burpees
- Jogging
- Yoga
- Basketball

You only need enough exercise to meet your own goals. Choose activities that fit your schedule, abilities, and needs. Start slowly, build up gradually, and stick with it.

6. Diet

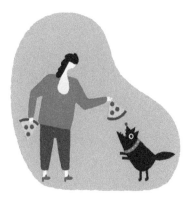

Your diet provides the chemicals your body needs to function, therefore what you eat is important as well as how you manage the stress that hunger creates. Often atypicals forget to eat and end up grabbing whatever is at hand or quickly stress eating. An inconsistent relationship with food might be part of the reason why atypicals are more likely to suffer from eating disorders.

We can avoid eating too much or too quickly by using smaller plates. That way, you're less likely to eat so quickly that your stomach can't catch up with your eyes. Chew slowly and enjoy the taste of the food.

Setting consistent mealtimes is important to eating regularly. Make meals a social occasion to ensure that they are a priority. Set lunch dates with co-workers or insist on family dinner as part of your routine. Incorporate breakfast into your morning ritual, even if it's just a smoothie.

A nutritionist and a food journal can help determine your diet's impact on your energy levels and ability to focus throughout the day. Record your diet in your treatment notebook for a few weeks and monitor the changes in your mood and energy levels.

Finally, keep in mind that your medication might affect your appetite. If you believe this is happening, bring it up with your prescribing clinician.

Brain stuff

Your brain is an 8-pound ball of grey fat that contains 100 billion neurons and controls everything you think and do. What you eat provides the construction and communication materials it needs to function. Three groups of micronutrients regulate communication between brain cells.

- *Minerals*: Magnesium, zinc, copper, iron, iodine, selenium, manganese, and potassium
- *Vitamins:* B6, B12, B3, and B9 (folate), E
- *Fatty acids*: Omega-3 and Omega-6

The best dietary sources of micronutrients are a topic of endless debate. You can find research to support almost any diet imaginable, so please do your own research. The following "good foods" and "bad foods" list works for me and, with the exception of animal proteins and vegetable oils, is fairly uncontroversial:

Foods with the good stuff

- Cruciferous vegetables (e.g. kale, collard greens, mustard greens, broccoli, sprouts, brussels sprouts, spinach)

- Legumes (e.g. black beans, chickpeas, kidney beans)

- Fruits (e.g. avocado, banana, raspberries, pineapple)

- Nuts and nut milks (e.g. walnuts, flaxseeds, peanuts, cashews, almonds, Brazil nuts, raw cacao)

- Fatty fish (e.g. salmon, mackerel, sardines)

- Whole grains (e.g. brown rice, whole grain oats, quinoa)

- Mushrooms

- Animal proteins (poultry, lamb, eggs, butter)

- Vegetable oils (e.g. olive, soybean, safflower, sunflower, corn, canola)

Bad foods

Recent studies have linked high-fat diets with brain inflammation and depression. Modern diets are the result of a cultural shift toward higher amounts of saturated fats and disproportionate amounts of Omega-6 due to increased consumption of dairy products, vegetable oils, and red meat. The negative impact of this change was further compounded by a reduction of fruits, vegetables, legumes, grains, and fish.

Fats that are solid at room temperature should mostly be avoided. Common sources of saturated fat include red meat, whole milk, cheese, coconut oil, and many commercially prepared baked goods. Other foods to be avoided include sugar, artificial colors, wheat products, aspartame, and alcohol.

7. Meditation

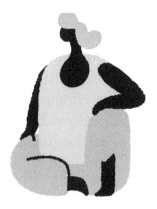

Meditation is a mindfulness exercise which helps manage thoughts and emotions. Meditation releases calming neuro-chemicals and trains your mind to more easily achieve a state of mental clarity and emotional stability.

There are many meditation techniques, but breathing is always the starting point. Breathing is much more powerful and important to the brain function than most people real-ize. It increases the oxygen available to your brain. Notice your breathing. You don't need to alter your breathing in any way, just observe the air moving in and out of your body. How long can you focus only on your breath before other thoughts intrude and pull you away? This is not an easy or trivial exercise. It is the first step toward taming the elephant of your mind.

Taming the Elephant

An elephant is very strong and could easily cause chaos, trampling your mental garden. But if you spend time training the elephant, you can ride it and it will help plow your fields. The elephant won't be trained in a single day, however. Your mind is that elephant and your conscious will is the rider.

The Train Station

"It is the mark of an educated mind to be able to entertain a thought without accepting it."

–Aristotle, Metaphysics

Now imagine that you are sitting on the platform in a train station. You are watching the trains come and go. The trains are thoughts passing through your mind and they are powered by your emotions. If you aren't careful, you unconsciously board almost every train. You ride it for a while before arbitrarily hopping aboard another. We spend our whole day racing around on these trains. But what if you didn't get on the trains? You don't need to.

Meditation helps you remain at the station. Observe the trains. Think about where they come from and where they are headed.

Then you can choose which trains to board and avoid expending energy on useless thoughts.

When you inevitably find yourself aboard a train by accident, remember that you can always get off and return to the station, that safe, centered place within yourself.

8. Physiological Treatment Plan

Create your own physiological treatment plan and mark off what you've done throughout the day on paper or with a task app. Be mindful of your natural biological rhythms to help make it easier to exercise, sleep, and maintain healthy eating habits. Finally, remember that your physiology can be enormously influenced by external forces like weather, temperature, seasons, life circumstances, screen time, stress, and recurring thoughts.

Below is an example template to help you get started tracking your daily physiological treatment. Record your activities and note treatment areas that need more attention as well as areas where you naturally succeed.

- *Medication:* 9am (x/x)
- *Sleep:* 10pm-6am (0/8 hours)
- *Exercise:* (x/60 minutes)
- *Diet:* (water x/8) (fruit x/6) meat (x/2) veg (x/5) grain (x/3) fish
- *Meditation:* x/15 minutes (x/2)
- *Mantra:* "I am doing better every day."

ADHD BEHAVIOR

Introduction

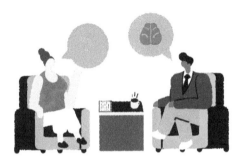

Behavioral treatments help you translate physiological improvements, such as greater focus, impulse control, and emotional centeredness, into meaningful actions. Behavioral treatments can be more difficult to implement than physiological treatments and success might be less clearly defined.

Marcus Aurelius said, "Your mind is dyed with the color of your thoughts." As you work on the treatments in this section, remember to embrace challenges and love yourself, no matter what circumstances arise.

1. Reprogramming

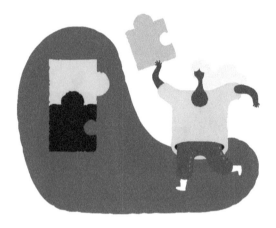

Reprogramming your habits and worldview is a lifelong process. You are the only one capable of helping you, and you already have everything you need. Positive results depend heavily on stress reduction. Pause, be aware, and recognize what change you'd like to make going forward. Then, you can take preemptive actions to minimize triggers and shape your reactions according to your values.

The emotional, cognitive, and behavioral obstacles you deal with are all a result of your current internal programming. These subconscious patterns were installed in early childhood and often go unexamined until we encounter problems because the patterns do not serve us anymore. It is impossible to change your programming without understanding it. Here is a list of tools that can help:

- Deep relaxation or meditation
- Deep breathing exercises
- Affirmations
- Visualizing success
- Sitting with your inner child
- Exploring your inner space
- Talking to your inner guardians
- Controlled emotional outbursts
- Self-hypnosis
- Therapy

Notice how your worldview is reinforced by the way you express yourself. Try to identify negative statements and rephrase the same information in a positive way. For example, rather than say, "I'm going through a hard time," or, "I'm depressed," you could say something hopeful and transformative like, "I'm getting better every day."

Write out your perfect day from start to finish. Compare the vision to your values. Are there some values missing due to limiting beliefs from your negativity? Are you avoiding paying attention to some values unintentionally? Create an aspirational, positive reality to be your destination.

My perfect day starts with:

_____

And then:

_____

And finally:

_____

Water flowers, not weeds

If your identity is a garden, choose to spend time watering your favorite flowers. People often spend time tending to flowers that they don't like because of external pressure from others.

2. Emotional Obstacles

Emotions are the source of behavior and our internal distraction. They flood us and overwhelm all reason or slowly drip and wear us down over time. It can feel as if emotions are uncontrollable—something that happens to you, like a rainstorm—but the truth is you create those emotions and you can control them. Or at least your reaction to them. Let's look at how to identify and treat the obstacles that emotions can create.

When a negative feeling arises, take notice but don't struggle. It is a part of you that arises in response to particular stimuli, like a mouse that pokes its head out of a hole when it smells food.

Don't panic. More stress will give energy to the feeling. Welcome the feeling and remind yourself that it will pass.

Don't ignore it. Instead, observe the feeling. Where do you feel it in your body? What are the qualities of the feeling?

Visualize it. Give it a shape, color, mass, texture, and smell.

Acknowledge the feeling and reassure it that you know what it wants to say in this moment. Then, explain that there are things you need to get done anyway and put it aside.

1. Acknowledge the feeling.

2. Label each emotion.

3. Determine triggers.

4. Relax and focus on what you can control.

5. Are you upset with yourself or someone else? Think about all sides.

6. Appropriately express your emotions and take some time for yourself.

7. Return to the situation when you are calm and resolve the emotion by talking to someone or reflecting.

It is easy to find evidence of your flaws and fall into a vicious cycle in which a jaded outlook leads to low expectations and poor performance. Low expectations of yourself naturally lead to poor outcomes.

Short-circuit those self-defeating ideas and replace them with self-supporting, grounded perspectives and pragmatic efforts to adapt. Don't give up when you fail; learn the lesson and seek creative solutions for next time. Create a mantra that diminishes the negative thoughts.

"OK, here's another challenge, just like the ones I've faced before. I am an expert in this type of thing. I have handled my share of these obstacles and I'm still standing. Let's do this."

Stress

Stress is your biggest obstacle because it pressures you into familiar, maladaptive patterns of behavior. Managing stress is a challenging, never-ending struggle. Be patient and compassionate with yourself because stress will flow over you and seep into all of your weak points.

Locate the stress in your body. Challenge the thoughts accompanying that feeling and separate fact from emotion. Are the stressful thoughts true? Will you let those thoughts and emotions control this moment? Could you step away from this pattern in a positive way rather than pursuing a familiar, negative spiral?

- Fear and panic only know how to say, "stop"
- Pause to breathe, challenge the feeling, and go forward

Shame

Shame is not a useful emotion. Shame tells us that, regardless of whether our actions are OK or not, who we are isn't. It is not resolvable because you can't change yourself.

Do you apologize too much? Feel misunderstood? Make self-deprecating comments? Have fragile self-esteem? Make excuses?

"Shame on you" is a curse people put on you. Shame paralyzes us. It stops us from acting. It blocks our creative energy and makes us doubt our inherent goodness. Many of us are taught from an early age to feel ashamed for having basic needs. Change the rules. You have the right to be successful and happy. You are enough.

If shame is trying to enforce a false or inappropriate message, change the message. If you can't change the message, surrender to the situation and love yourself anyway.

Separate yourself from your bad behavior and challenge the shame. You can't change the past, but you can forgive yourself. There are no fresh starts, but there are always opportunities to do better.

Self-blame

ADHD is a medical condition. No one asks for or wants these symptoms. A lifetime of feeling unsuccessful and failing to meet expectations can become an emotional obstacle that prevents self-improvement. It's death by a thousand cuts:

- "Things will never work out for me."
- "I'm a mess."
- "Why do I always get stuck like this?"
- "I should have started earlier."
- "What's wrong with me?"
- "Everyone must think I'm stupid."

ADHD symptoms damage self-esteem. We blame ourselves rather than our ADHD. Self-blame makes us feel stuck and helpless because we can't change ourselves. It is a waste of time.

Are you often self-critical? Do you often appear overwhelmed or demoralized?

Do you tend to talk about life in a negative, hopeless manner?

Love yourself and challenge your condition. It's not easy, but you can redirect your emotional energy to stop blaming yourself and start challenging problematic behaviors.

Grief

Mourning lost opportunities. The anguish of failure. Self-pity for needing to work twice as hard just to keep up. Notice your grief and allow it to happen. Get some outside perspectives from a therapist, close friends, or family members.

Understand the child you were when you first began to experience these feelings. That child couldn't understand their condition or its implications. Living with a burden they weren't even aware of, and all the emotional trauma that came with it. That child was just trying to survive. See your history in a new, compassionate light. Put the past into a new context. You are an adult now. You can love that child and make informed choices.

Enjoy the experience of discovering your true potential, no matter what age. Stop beating yourself up. Creating a positive self-narrative is easier said than done. You might need to be effective before you feel effective. Keep working on it, be proud of your past self, and celebrate your recent wins.

The way you think will determine your future successes, therefore it is critical to let go of grief and accept who you are. Comparing yourself to others only causes misery.

Dread

At some point, you probably started dreading certain things, like job interviews, because you didn't understand what was going wrong or how your unconscious behaviors and symptoms led to failure. Understanding your condition puts these patterns into a new context. Get excited about the activities you learned to dread because now you can approach them with a clear understanding of your strengths and weaknesses.

Fatigue

Atypicals expend a lot of energy managing everyday tasks that others take for granted. Tasks neurotypicals can do on autopilot are not so easy for us.

Protect your focus and eliminate emotional energy drains from your life. Designate a "safe" friend to check in with when you are overwhelmed and reject toxic relationships. Use positive self-talk to pump yourself up. Don't make assumptions. Get the facts. No one can read your mind and you can't read minds either. Take five. Identify your anger, fear, or desire to withdraw. Express your feelings calmly. Write it down if it helps. Talk to a therapist.

3. Cognitive Obstacles

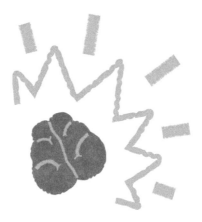

Emotions lead to thoughts and sometimes those thoughts are self-critical or negative. Everyone experiences negative thinking from time to time, but persistent negative thoughts can distort your interpretation of reality. Avoid destructive patterns of thinking by recognizing and challenging them with real facts.

Cognitive distortions (ANTs)

Recurring cognitive distortions are sometimes called ANTs (automatic negative thoughts). One ANT is a minor irritation, but if you don't deal with them, you will quickly be overwhelmed. Examples of ANTs to look out for are listed with examples below:

Overgeneralizing

Assuming that everything happens a certain way and ignoring information. Applying the outcome of one experience to every experience. A single negative event is seen as an unavoidable pattern:

- "I never complete anything."
- "There's nothing to do."
- "I'm the worst at this."
- "If I fail at this, I'm no good at anything."
- "This always happens."
- "Everyone hates me."
- "You never listen to me."

Personalizing

Blaming yourself for another person's actions:

- "She didn't ask me to lead the project because she knows I'd screw it up."

Catastrophizing

Mentally building up a minor difficulty into a major catastrophe:

- "If I bomb this test, my life is over."

Mind reading

Assuming you know what people are thinking and why. Don't try to read people's thoughts; most people don't know what they're thinking and are mostly too busy thinking about themselves to spend time thinking about you:

- "She complimented my friend, which means she doesn't like me."

Self-fulfilling prophecy

Assuming you know the future and that it will be bad. You may think you're preparing yourself–protecting yourself in advance–but you're actually pointing yourself toward failure. When you predict bad things, they do become more likely. Don't let irrational fears guide your thoughts:

- "This is about to go badly."
- "People will laugh at me."

Magnification or minimization

You exaggerate the importance of problems and minimize your strengths:

- "Without my lucky pencil there's no way I can pass this test."

Self-shaming

Believing that you're not good enough. Shame uses words such as "should," "must," "ought to," or "have to." Whenever we think we must do something, we don't want to do it. That's human nature.

- "I should be better at this."
- "I'm the reason our team failed to make the goal."

Change those phrases to "I want to," "It fits my goals to," "It would be helpful to," "It's in my best interest to."

Labeling

Negative labels are very harmful. When you attach a label to something you sabotage your ability to see it clearly. People label others to avoid doing the work of understanding them. They simply decide to always expect the worst.

- Lazy, dummy, idiot, failure, spoiled brat, careless, clown

Blame

Blaming other people for your problems to avoid accountability. Blaming others makes you powerless to change anything. It never helps. Take responsibility to change the problems you have.

- "I told you this was a bad idea…"
- "That wouldn't have happened if you had…"

Negative lens

You focus on the bad and ignore the good. When you need to leave, you only think of what is being left behind, not the cool things ahead. Don't assume your negative worldview accurately reflects reality. Feelings are complicated and often meaningless. Don't rely on them to make decisions.

- "Life sucks."

Crushing ANTs

Learn to recognize ANTs and crush them before they cause problems. When you have ANTs, examine them and look for evidence of the truth. Do you have real reasons to feel this way, or are your feelings based on events from the past? The past is over and it does not control the future.

You have probably spent years repeating and reinforcing your ANTs. They can start to feel like a part of your identity and worldview. They might even be reinforced by your family. Examine your social circle and make changes in your life to ensure a positive and supportive social environment.

Quick, defusing comments and self-awareness can help. "There I go again, thinking I can predict the future." Be kind to yourself. These things are difficult and take time to change.

4. Behavioral Obstacles

Think about why you feel like you can't do it. If you feel like you can't start, you haven't made the task small enough.

A combination of emotions and thoughts are responsible for our behavior. Certain behaviors prevent meaningful action. We are paralyzed by fear or distraction. The following tips address some of the maladaptive behaviors that are common trouble spots for atypicals.

Procrastination

Procrastination isn't about avoiding work. It's about avoiding feelings. Success or failure will bring changes, embarrassment, or increased responsibilities. It is the desire to avoid those unknowns which causes you to procrastinate. Putting off a task feels immediately rewarding and avoids the fear of potentially threatening upheaval. Success or failure may change people's expectations of you, your view of yourself, or your circumstances.

Your view of feedback is critical. Successful people take criticism as constructive. Unsuccessful people view criticism as personal rejection, a permanent fixture of their identity, which prevents them from moving forward.

Curiosity about what you are afraid of will help extinguish the paralyzing fears which cause procrastination. What fear is sabotaging your efforts to move forward?

Types of procrastination and solutions

- Ineffective prioritizing

  Problem: Only attending to tasks of interest.

  Solution: Create and stick to a well-laid plan. Focus on the emotional endpoint.

- Forgetfulness

  Problem: Insufficient working memory.

  Solution: Repetition, consistency, and stress reduction. Visual reminders of the plan.

- Distracted

  Problem: Something else comes up.

Solution: Structures to screen distractions and rewards for task completion. Timers for short, focused sprints.

- Overwhelmed

  Problem: Tasks seem to be an overwhelming whole.

  Solution: Chunk tasks into manageable pieces.

- Perfectionism

  Problem: Unusually high standards and fear of failure.

  Solution: Lower the stakes. Put it in perspective. Set time limits and incentives.

Perfectionism

Demanding perfection is a great excuse for never finishing a task, thereby avoiding anxiety. Perfectionism is the fear that you're not enough combined with the self-delusion that you are special. "I'm special, therefore my work must be flawless."

Don't let perfectionism waste your time. Remember, if something is worth doing, it's worth doing poorly. Striving for perfectionism forces you to sacrifice everything else. "It's OK if this is not my best work as long as it satisfies the requirements. "This work is not a reflection of my value as a person. I will do the best I can with the time I have." Done is better than perfect.

Future nearsighted

Atypicals tend to be oblivious to the future and underestimate how long things take. Improving your ability to think ahead, estimate how long things take, and deliver on deadlines, are vital skills for atypicals to work on. Consistent use of your calendar and the other critical treatment tools can help with this.

Popcorn thoughts

Thoughts constantly pop into our head out of nowhere. Unfortunately, the difficulty we have with prioritizing information means new information is automatically prioritized. This quickly becomes overwhelming. When thoughts pop up, write them in your treatment notebook and deal with them during your evening check-in.

The power of the first thing

Set up your day with positive behaviors. Challenge yourself to put off familiar distractions, like checking social media, for longer and longer each day. Putting off that first indulgence builds the muscle needed to overcome distraction.

Think about the first time each day that you give into a temptation and put off your best intentions. Your first indulgence makes subsequent indulgences easier. "Well, today is already wasted, so I might as well..." This type of thinking is a self-defeating trap. A few slip-ups don't mean the day is wasted. Remember the consequences of pursuing the same empty loop in the past and do better.

5. Awareness

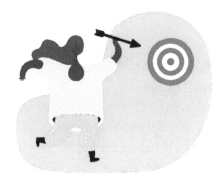

Awareness is a sense of present mindfulness that helps us act with conscious intention from moment to moment. It's how we recognize our values and what we love about being alive. It is not a talent, but a skill that you strengthen. Awareness helps you to maintain a positive attitude, acknowledge your strengths, and identify distractions. It starts with making time for honest reflection and self-assessment.

More benefits of awareness

- Discover your values
- Identify your strengths and weaknesses

- Maintain a positive attitude and a desire to improve
- Separate your behavior from your self
- Repair self-esteem
- Accept feedback from your treatment team
- Monitor and limit your distractions
- Monitor your wellness and self-care routinely

Examine your outlook

Success, Happiness, Fulfillment

Think about the associations and assumptions you have about each of these words. What comes up? Write it down. Don't take your truth for granted; it impacts your entire perspective and ability to make different choices.

People could be thinking negative or positive thoughts about you at every moment. You'll never know. You get to decide which of those worlds you live in.

Step over the line and enter the more positive world. Make a Yes/No board. What thoughts will you say yes and no to moving forward?

The helicopter

Picture your life as if you were watching yourself from a helicopter. What would you notice about your routines? How do you choose to spend time compared to your ideals?

Inner child

Talk to your child self about specific circumstances of your life. How would your child self feel about these things? Understand what caused your perspective and examine it.

You need to examine and reprocess past trauma to make room for a new worldview.

Ask your child self, "What are you afraid of?" "How do you protect yourself?" Then, ask your present self, "Do those behaviors still serve me?"

Inner guardian

Imagine three people (guardians) that you could count on to always protect you and give you positive encouragement. They can be real or fictional. Your best friend, a great philosopher, or a superhero are all potential choices. I chose Marcus Aurelius, Winnie the Pooh, and Mr. Rogers. When you consider past trauma–situations that would have caused confusion, fear, or shame for your child self–consider what your guardians would say to that child.

Inner castle

Close your eyes and construct a room inside your mind. Somewhere you are safe to do anything you want. A place that's free of any external pressure. No one can come in this room unless you invite them in. When you panic, remember that this room is always here for you. As you return to this place, you might even notice additional rooms, which you rarely visit. Don't be afraid to explore; these are all safe spaces.

Emotional outburst therapy

Lie on your back on a bed and kick your arms and legs. Go deep into the forest and scream. Yell into a pillow. Watch a movie that makes you cry.

Under appropriate circumstances, an emotional outburst can be as necessary and relaxing to your emotional self as exercise is to your physical self.

Perspective and choice

New perspectives can help you become aware of how you are stuck, what beliefs you are stubbornly defending. Always look for new choices you can make. Choice gives us power and fulfillment. Winners move and attack while victims defend and react. Don't live in constant retreat from life. Look at your worldview and see more of the available choices. How would your inner guardian look at this situation? What advice would they give?

When we're stressed, and our impulsivity takes over, we aren't mindful. In those moments, it often feels as if we know right from wrong, but choose wrong anyway. Make a list of things you never want to do, say, think, or feel. Conscious thoughts are just the tip of the iceberg. You might consciously want to do something, but unconsciously want not to do it; unrecognized internal contradictions can easily sink your best intentions.

Develop an internal awareness monitor. "How do I know when I am fully present?" "What am I choosing right now?" "Where is my awareness?" Meditation is a good way to train your awareness muscle.

6. Thought & Emotion Record

Keep a record of thoughts and emotions in your notebook or use a mood tracking app to identify cycles of thought or emotion.

Write about a recent situation that upset you. Note what you were thinking and feeling at the time. What were you saying about the situation and your role in it?

Now ask yourself, could this have happened to anyone? Was it out of your control? Were there factors that made the problem hard to avoid?

Now think about what you realistically could have done to avoid the situation.

Finally, come up with a useful statement to tell yourself next time a similar situation occurs. It might help to imagine what one of your friends or inner guardians would say about it.

7. Mantras

Mantras are powerful, self-affirming statements that help recenter your focus and shake off negative thoughts. Observe your recurrent negative thoughts, then think of a positive mantra that subverts them. Repeat it to yourself when those thoughts return.

A mantra that makes you smile with its humor and compassion defuses negativity. "Here's my foolishness again. Nothing that I haven't faced before. I fear nothing. I regret nothing. I am an unstoppable force." Be proud of yourself for recognizing your fears and insecurities. Laugh at them.

Example mantras

- It's OK to be who I am.
- I am lovable and I can love. I am enough.
- I don't need to do anything special.
- I never need to apologize for being myself.

Fill yourself with positive thoughts, and there will be no room for negative thoughts. Be proud of yourself for recognizing your challenges and making efforts to overcome them.

8. Remembering

Forgetting something does not mean you didn't care enough to remember.

Atypicals struggle to recall specific information at the right moment. We fail to remember appointments, where we put our keys, or that the laundry needs to be done. The tips below will help strengthen your ability to access relevant information and avoid being blindsided by the consequences of forgetting.

Pause

Pause and give an experience the attention it requires in order to form a lasting memory. Pause and consider what you might be forgetting, what else could be done, and how this will affect others. Panic and haste are the enemies of memory. A pause to breathe helps you calm down, appreciate details, and make vivid memories.

Repetition

Emotions, repetition, and novelty solidify memories. Repeat what you need to do three times. Ask yourself questions. Describe things you need to remember. Reflect on the emotions of what has happened.

Write it down

Writing clarifies and contextualizes memories. Use a section of your treatment notebook as a journal or diary. It's not real until it's written.

Sensory visualization

Use multiple senses. Focus on the feeling of the pill on your tongue to help you remember that you've taken your meds. Smell everything.

We think in pictures. Make a picture of what you want to remember in your mind. Focus on the details with each of your senses.

You can strengthen sensory associations through practice. Examine an object, noting the details, then put it away and recreate it in your mind with your eyes closed.

Visualization is also helpful for memorizing sequences. Rehearse the steps of a process in your mind and there will be one less obstacle when it comes time to actually do it.

Novel association

Associate the information you want to remember with other things. Park in a spot where you need to squeeze in next to a support beam and associate the parking spot with the beam.

Hook new information onto something else

When you learn someone's name, associate it with a word that begins with the same letter (Larry - lamb) or a rhyming word (Shawn - pawn). Novel associations create vivid imagery with the new information, making it easier to recall. If something is interesting, notable, or engaging, it is easier to keep in mind.

Method of Loci

Visualize the things you need to remember as objects, then imagine yourself placing the objects around a room. The room could be a familiar place or totally imaginary. *The Method of Loci* relies on spatial relationships and objects as memory hooks. For example, you could put your upcoming therapy appointment on the green couch. Put your to-do list on the small table next to the flickering lamp. You could even go to different rooms to put different types of information.

Long-term memory

Keeping track of things requires short-term memory, but atypicals often don't make a short-term memory in the first place. Relying more on long-term memory can help circumvent some of the problems caused by this issue. Have a time and place for everything. Do certain things at certain times. Have a little home for each item in your house, car, and bag. Your routines, launchpad, traveling checklist, and alarms can help you establish long-term memories. Be consistent.

Routines

New routines take a long time to learn, they feel awkward, and are easy to avoid. No one said it would be easy. As you approach the task of installing a new routine, be aware of the challenges and you will be ready to overcome them. Your goal is to make healthy routines so unavoidable that they become habits, but don't count on that happening quickly.

Rely on your visual reminders, checklists, and timers. Rely on the structure they provide to decrease the stress of forgetting.

9. Building Confidence

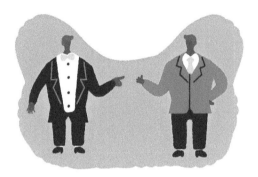

Do things you're good at regularly and believe in yourself no matter what. Recognize the unavoidable and often frustrating challenges of learning something new. Know your limits and you'll be less likely to become frustrated by failing at a difficult task. Finally, if something comes easily to you, it is not because you did it wrong or because that thing is easy for everyone. Give yourself credit and reward small victories.

Outsource encouragement

Sometimes we get into the habit of avoiding asking others for help. Rely on your treatment team for things you struggle with. They provide accountability with reality checks about self-care, your strengths and weaknesses, and overall progress. Ask for feedback. What do they see?

Remember, you wouldn't tell someone that taking insulin to treat their diabetes was a crutch. ADHD is a real biological condition, not something you can overcome with willpower alone. Feeling like you need to conquer ADHD without any external help is a recipe for failure and self-shaming.

10. Motivation & Intention

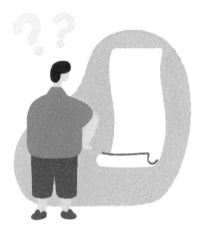

Motivation is the willingness or desire to activate forethought, engage, and commit sustained effort toward completing a task. Motivation is a fundamental struggle for atypicals. You can learn to self-motivate, but it will likely take more effort than your neurotypical peers.

Emotion is the key to motivation. What do you want? How does that fulfill your values and sense of purpose?

Focus on the positive emotions—the joy of attainment—and use them as motivation to get started.

You need to care

We can get demoralized into feeling like our future doesn't offer much. Nihilism is poison. Nothing inherently matters, but everyone needs something that matters to them personally. You get to choose. Identify your drives and psych yourself up like an athlete. Build energy through focused breathing, light exercise, or visualization of the emotional high you will experience upon completing your objective.

The power of choice

Remember that no one is forcing you to do anything. You get to make the choice to improve your life:

- Celebrate the joy and power of pursuing your wants.
- Choose the right environment.
- Choose music that will pump you up.
- Choose your tasks and accountability structure.
- Choose your rewards.

11. Prioritizing

It feels as if there is a red light in my head that flashes whenever a new stimulus enters my awareness. My brain is like a beehive that gets tapped on, prompting all my thought bees to scramble around on high alert for a few minutes. It doesn't matter what the stimulus is; a phone rings, a bad smell, an email hits my inbox. Literally anything that I experience becomes a priority that must be assessed before returning to the task at hand.

It can also be difficult to determine which one of my important tasks is most important without becoming overwhelmed. Use the tips below to manage priorities more effectively.

Palette cleanser

What's your preferred beverage to wash a bad taste out of your mouth? Find a quick action that can help you reset and resume your intended activity. Observe what helps you shake off distractions quickly. A few push-ups, a walk, or just an acknowledgment that your attention was briefly hijacked. Discover what puts your mind back on track.

Stick to the plan

Make a plan during your evening check-in and stick to the plan. Ignore the stimuli that pop up and demand your attention throughout the day. Those things can be written down and scheduled at a more appropriate time. Getting sidetracked might seem like nimble multitasking, but it derails your momentum toward the ultimate objective. This is why you have a plan.

White-knuckle it.

Make criteria

Having criteria for prioritizing tasks and items can make the process more efficient and manageable. Prioritize everything with a letter to signify its level of urgency and importance:

- **A-Tier** items are urgent and important. They are time-sensitive and vital to advancing your goals. *Bills or work tasks.*

- **B-Tier** items are important but not urgent. They don't need to be done today. *Updating your mailing address or going on a date.*

- **C-Tier** is for items that are interesting but not important or urgent. *Things that you'd like to get to in the next few months. Things on your bucket list.*

Once your tasks are sorted into tiers A, B, or C you can assign them a number to indicate the order each task should be completed. A-tasks must be completed before B-tasks and A1 needs to be done before A2.

12. Goals

Before making a plan, you need clear goals. Whether its life goals, monthly milestones, or daily tasks, the components are the same. Use the SMART goal structure to set effective goals so you are prepared to make a plan with straightforward steps.

SMART goals

"I want to be more organized," is too vague to be useful. The sentiment is admirable, but without specific deliverables and deadlines, the process lacks clarity. What exactly will you do to be organized? That is part of the goal. Atypicals have great ideas but have difficulty sustaining effort and following through consistently. Be as specific as possible about where, when, how long, and how much.

Make your goals SMART goals:

- **Specific** - What exactly will you accomplish?
- **Measurable** - How will you know when it is accomplished?

- **Achievable** - Is it realistic that you can accomplish the goal based on available resources like time, skill, and materials?

- **Relevant** - Does accomplishing this goal advance my greater interests?

- **Time-based** - How long will this take?

What are you saying 'yes' to by pursuing these goals? What meaningful purpose could you fulfill by achieving these goals? What needs to change inside to create change outside?

13. Planning

Planning is the key to reliably achieving your goals. Use the following tips to help you make plans that work and result in outcomes that improve your life.

Set a meeting with yourself for planning

Prioritize and protect your planning time. Take it as seriously as a meeting with another person. It is that important. Set an alarm to remember this important meeting. Plan, then plan to remember.

Planning checklist

- Why am I doing this? What result do I desire?
- Is the next step clear and vivid in my mind?
- Am I internally distracted?
- Is my environment distracting?

Plan in reverse

Plan backward from the deadline until you find the start time. Adding an additional cushion of time helps avoid stress. The future exists, so plan to do a little bit each day. Once you have a SMART goal in mind, create a plan to follow through:

- Break the goal down into its simplest component tasks.

- Set a deadline for the goal.

- Make a plan to complete each component task.

- Locate necessary information.

- Anticipate setbacks.

- Consider several alternative ways you might achieve your goal.

- Take into account your strengths and weaknesses.

- Execute the tasks.

- Evaluate how well the plan worked.

Problems that interfere with planning

Do you get sidetracked while doing tasks? Does your mind feel busy or clouded? Are you daydreaming? Are you thinking about the other things you need to do right now?

- *Lack of clear plans:* Chaos is distracting. We need structure and limits to move efficiently toward a destination.

- *Internal distractions:* Physical, emotional, pace, stress

- *External distractions:* Uncontrollable sensory stimuli

14. Progress

Reflect on your progress routinely in order to maintain motivation and increase your efficacy.

Review last week's goals. If goals were met, think about why you were able to succeed and how you were rewarded. What helped you follow through? What prevented you from following through? Did you reward yourself? Focus on accomplishments and approach failed objectives as learning experiences. Record observations in your treatment notebook about what motivates your progress.

Momentum

Any route, well-traveled, becomes easier. Build momentum by staying in motion. Defuse fear with curiosity and celebrate small victories.

15. Play

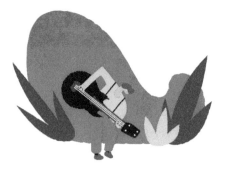

Play is purposeless fun with no end goal. Play is voluntary curiosity and experimentation that possesses an inherent attraction. When we are playing, we are not self-conscious. Although play does not have a fixed purpose, it is essential to learning. Play teaches us problem-solving, independence, socialization, analysis, understanding of rules, etc. Imagination and daydreaming are internal forms of play.

Fun menu

When we become stressed, fun is often the first thing to go. Sometimes it's difficult to even think of the activities we enjoy.

To make it easier, create a fun menu, listing things that bring you joy.

Little delights

Add things to your day that make you feel more playful: clothes, music, art on the wall. Even forcing a smile, dancing, or singing a song can provide a little emotional boost. What little things make you happy (explore all five senses) that you can add to your day?

Schedule fun first

When you make your calendar, schedule fun things first. This approach places emphasis on the things you are looking forward to, so even when things are tough, there's light at the end of the tunnel.

Relaxation

Keep in mind that fun is different from relaxation. Fun is stimulating, while relaxation is restful. You need both fun and relaxation.

Gamify tasks

We grow up learning to play, then we are reprogrammed to work. You can use your natural inclination for play to make boring tasks more enjoyable. Try implementing a point system, rewards, or a race against the clock for tasks you dread.

16. Personal Style

Identity

What is your identity and how do you express it? We judge others by their physical appearance and bearing. The things we can control about our appearance include our clothes, hygiene, and presence. Many atypicals learn to hide their identities and eschew personal style as an unconscious reaction to years of enforced conformity and criticism.

Clothing

- Do you have self-esteem issues that make you avoid thinking about clothes?

- Are there fabrics you prefer to wear? Loose or fitted? Colorful or monochrome?

- Do you know your sizes?

My uniform

Think of your "uniform," the type of outfit that suits you 90% of the time. This helps diminish decision fatigue. Your brain has the energy for a certain number of decisions in a single day. Don't waste them. Use a minimalist palette. Keep it simple.

The Hanger Trick

Consider what you actually wear. Try the hanger trick to keep track of what you actually wear in a month. Just put all your hangers facing one direction, then turn them after you wear the item that hangs on it. After a few weeks, you'll be able to identify what you never wear. Keep a record of outfits that work. Get rid of things you don't wear.

Hygiene

Cleanliness is next to godliness. Your body and your clothes must be clean and smell pleasant. Look at yourself in the mirror as if you were deciding whether to hire that person. Hygiene also includes any hair and makeup considerations.

Presence

How you carry yourself and interact with others is the most important factor in how people treat you. Presence is characterized mostly by non-verbal cues that communicate your status to others. It tells others how you expect to be treated. Humans are constantly thinking about their status in relation to others.

Here are some examples of status cues:

- Do you exude calm or anxious energy?

- Are your movements deliberate and steady or fidgety and quick?

- Do you perform tasks with workmanlike efficiency or obvious labor?

- Is your posture expansive or contractive?

- Are you non-reactive and steadfast or are you either compliant or hyper-reactive?

Good posture and a calm demeanor put others at ease and also has physiological benefits. Think of improvements to your general bearing as a form of low-impact exercise.

17. Creativity

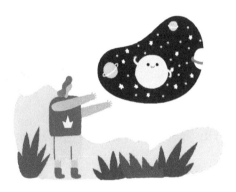

Atypicals are divergent thinkers. Our minds take an indirect route from A to B, discovering hidden treasures and unexpected connections along the way. Atypicals experience a broad range of emotions and intuitively impart those feelings into their creations.

Unfortunately, our ability to create is often hampered by our symptoms. Hyperfocus can be beneficial, but is offset by short attention and impaired working memory, which makes communicating sustained thoughts difficult. Hypersensitivity to criticism and rejection can also cause us to become ashamed of our creativity and self-sabotage in the absence of sufficient encouragement.

External factors also converge to dampen our creative spirit. Our culture does not value or accommodate creativity except in a productive, manufacturing sense.

Atypicals learn by doing, but most education systems are designed to teach by thinking rather than doing; lots of reading and talking, but little hands-on experience. The poor fit between mainstream education and ADHD learning styles can result in low self-esteem, an unsatisfactory education, and lingering trauma.

Creativity myths

- Creativity has little value in the work-a-day world.
- Creative people can't make a good living.
- Creative people are troublemakers.
- Creative ways are not efficient.
- You can't be creative and responsible.
- Creative people are not grounded.
- Creative thinking is not as good as linear ways of doing things.
- Creativity has no structure or form.
- It's no big deal to be creative because children or anyone can do it.
- You can't be creative unless you have a special talent.

As our creativity is damaged or severed from us, we grieve. We tell ourselves that, "My creativity is not important anyway." We cover our grief with anger. We comfort ourselves with fantasies about pursuing our creativity later in life, perhaps in retirement. Finally, we become depressed and force ourselves to forget why. You don't need to accept the loss of your creativity, and it is possible to reconnect with it.

Rediscovering creativity

"Shoulds" do not reflect your authentic self; "wants" do. Reconnecting with your creativity means getting in touch with your wants. After ignoring them for many years, this process might require an external trigger. A life change. An unexpected opportunity to reconnect.

Listen to your inner feelings and allow yourself to be creative without self-criticism. Visualize the child inside you who was told not to be creative and encourage them. It's safe now.

Explore your creative identity, build creative competence, and enjoy the emotional connection you develop with your creations. Enjoy the value you have and appreciate the value of other people.

18. Behavioral Tactic Recap

We've covered a lot of behavioral tactics which will help over-come some of the problematic behavior caused by your symptoms. Below are a few tactics to review as you consider what might benefit your treatment efforts:

- Who are you when you love yourself most?

- Date yourself. Learn your wants and try to impress yourself.

- Kill ANTs.

- Make soft commitments. Recognize that, when you say "yes," you are saying "no" to other possibilities.

- Accept the uncontrollable.

- It's never the perfect time and there are no fresh starts.

- Observe your emotions and challenge your thoughts.

- Be compassionate with your past and ambitious with your future.

- Build resilience by accepting failure and periods of sadness.

- Identify your energy rhythms.

- Practice relaxation exercises like steady breathing.

- Give thanks.

19. Behavioral Treatment Plan

Choose a recurring emotion that you'd like to diminish. How could you challenge this emotion when it returns? Is it valid? What triggers it?

- Emotion:
- Challenge:

Choose a recurring thought you'd like to diminish. How could you challenge this thought when it returns? Is it valid? What triggers it?

- Thought:
- Challenge:

Choose a recurring pattern of behavior you'd like to diminish. How could you challenge this thought when it returns? Is it valid? What triggers it? How would you like to respond instead?

- Behavior:
- Alternate behavior:

Now try the exercise with emotions, thoughts, and patterns of behavior you'd like to increase.

ADHD HOME

Introduction

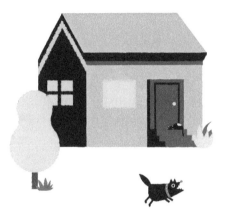

Home is an extension of your mind and a reflection of your relationship with yourself, a place that feels safe and enshrines your values. Who you are at home is the clearest reflection of who you can be at your best. At home, you are more able to control stress than anywhere else. If you share your home with others, then the reflection is influenced by those relationships and values as well. Take control of your home environment and push the limit of your potential.

1. Responsibilities

The first step to taking control of your home environment is to understand your responsibilities in this area. Understanding your home responsibilities makes it possible to schedule important tasks and refine the environment to diminish distractions and enhance your strengths.

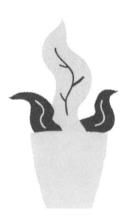

Home Responsibilities

- Emergency preparedness
- Personal finances
- Insurance and security
- Transportation
- Entertainment and electronics
- Health and cleanliness
- Childcare

- Friendship and romance
- Spiritual and intellectual growth
- Recreation

2. Environment

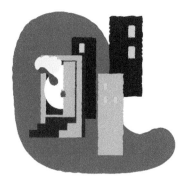

The right environment is critical to sticking with good routines. It can complement strengths, diminish distractions, and provide accountability. Bruce Wayne lives in a mansion, but underneath that is the bat cave. He divides his home in order to optimize each part for his different responsibilities. The visual cues are very different and enable him to think and behave differently. This is an extreme example, but demonstrates the importance and malleability of the stimuli in your home environment.

Monitor patterns in your emotions, actions, and energy levels to understand the triggers provided by your environment. If it's not working for you, change it. This is the one space where that is entirely acceptable. In your home it's either a "hell yeah" or a flat "no." What's your unique and beautiful life? Control the controllable.

3. Organization

Organization is a constant process that is never complete. Wash the dishes; they get dirty. Make dinner; it gets eaten. Sweep the floor, but there's always more dirt. Don't waste time trying to make things perfectly organized or punishing yourself for less than perfect. Done is better than perfect.

Benefits of getting organized

- Less material clutter = Less mental clutter
- More time for enjoyable activities
- Less overwhelmed about losing and finding things
- Better health
- Enjoy coming home and feeling accomplished and put together

In sight

Store items nearby where you will use them and keep frequently used items at eye level.

Organization buddy

An organization buddy might be able to help you sort through piles of stuff and give perspective about what's actually important. ADHD brains have trouble prioritizing, and an unbiased pair of eyes can be invaluable. Even simply imagining what a compassionate friend would say can help you make better decisions sometimes.

Wardrobe

- Organize your closet by clothing type.

- Does it fit? Is it sentimental? Will you need it in the future?

- How would you like people to think of you? Consider how your appearance can reflect this.

- Do your closet and dresser have an organizational structure?

4. Clutter

Some amount of clutter might be tolerable, but it usually harms everything else you do: your efficiency, your self-image, and your reputation with others. Consider the negative impacts clutter and disorganization might have on your life.

Visual clutter

Visual clutter creates stress and saps energy. Piles of stuff are often dismissed as your "quirky filing system," but they represent indecision, procrastination, and impulsivity. Set standards for cleanliness at home. Remove distractions and keep your space clean.

Spot cleaning

Spend 10 minutes at the end of each day doing spot cleaning. Set times for recurring organizational tasks like laundry. Place small containers in each room for "out of place" items.

Divide the space

A large task is overwhelming until you break it down. Start by focusing on one corner of a room. Set a timer for a short sprint, five or ten minutes, and commit to organizing that corner. Work clockwise around the room, focusing on small areas, then proceed that way through the other rooms. Resist the temptation to ignore the timer and hyperfocus; you don't want to spend all day on this and get burned out. After all, organizing is necessary, but it isn't *doing*. Take a break and reward yourself after each room is organized.

Clutter decision

When the moment comes, do you add to the clutter, or put things in their proper place? Declutter without shame or emotion. You don't need any of this junk to survive and it saps the energy required to do things you actually care about.

When sorting through clutter, don't hold onto anything for more than three seconds. Am I using it or is it trash? Keep moving, and don't second-guess. Remember the acronym, OHIO, which stands for "Only Handle It Once."

Holding onto papers represents indecisiveness. Decide what to do with each of your papers. Take action on it, put it into your organized filing system, or throw it away. Remember, OHIO. When in doubt, throw it out.

Organizing your papers

A file cabinet with labeled tabs can help store papers quickly and keep them easily accessible. Your file cabinet is not a storage bin to throw every loose paper into. Make categories for each of the things you want to hold onto: Education, Finances, Hobbies, Vision Board, etc.

One section of your filing system should be used as a "transit" or "action" file that you can remove and take with you to do errands right away. Sort these papers by their urgency and importance; things you need to do right away should come first. Reserve a special place for the action file and consider using a brightly-colored folder and it will be easier to remember.

Finally, keep a separate file for goals and projects. Add photos that remind you of your ideal future. Sensory visualization of rewards is what gets your inner manager excited to organize your life around. Review the items in the goal folder at least monthly.

Items

When you keep items you no longer use, they become damaged or destroyed. They become clutter. Use it or get rid of it.

- *Give it away* → Who could use those old items? Give it to them.

- *Replace it* → If you get something new, get rid of something old.

- *Store it* → Clear plastic bins with labels are like the filing cabinet of non-paper stuff.

- *Toss it* → Consider Marie Kondo's qualifying question, "Does it spark joy?" Throw the rest away.

The magic bin

If you invite guests over and want to put away the clutter in your house, get a bin with a lid and toss everything from your tabletops, counters and the floor into it before they arrive. The room will be clean and you can take out all the clutter again after they leave. You might even realize you didn't need any of that stuff after all.

Mental clutter

Keep your life roles separate in your mind to avoid carrying thoughts from one to another. Compartmentalize your thoughts so that you are always fully present and engaged.

Digital clutter

Desktop icons, unused apps, and social media notifications keep you checking your phone and diminish your focus. Clean it out. Turn off notifications, delete old contacts, and unused apps. Set your phone to silent and the colors to grayscale. Make your phone less fun.

5. Losing Things

When you lose something, don't allow your emotions to overwhelm your reason. Keep it in perspective; this happens to everyone. Reassure yourself that you will find the lost item and that worrying is not useful. Retrace your steps and know when it's time to take a break.

Stress causes carelessness

You are more likely to misplace things when you are stressed or distracted because it prevents you from giving important items sufficient attention. When you set down something important, note the objects next to it and their color. Anything that can associate your important object with the location. Novel association also works for remembering where you parked.

Make a list of what you lose most often and why. What would be the most annoying items to lose?

Common reasons for losing things

- You are stressed.

- You are late for something.

- You got distracted by something.

- You didn't use a list to help you remember.

- You write down important information in random places.

- You are multitasking

Electronic trackers

These little tiles are great for keeping track of keys and other easily misplaced items.

Make copies

Make copies or get a duplicate of anything you might lose easily, like keys and important information. Keep these things in consistent places.

6. Chores

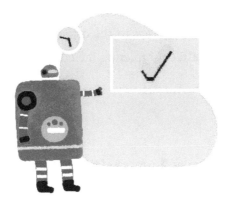

Getting started

Take some time to observe your home environment and listen to yourself. What would make you feel good if it was improved? Focus on the feeling of satisfaction. Use that to motivate you to get started.

Task circuits

If you have several tasks, you can complete them in circuits. For example, choose three chores and do a work sprint on each in rotation. Set a time limit for the chores and timers for the short sprints. Be careful not to hyperfocus on a single task, because you want the big reward of finishing. The future exists and there will be time to return to this task. Focus on small rewards and gradual progress.

Avoid pursuing every passing fancy by making a plan with specific tasks. Don't chastise yourself when you realize that you've wandered away. Just like when you are driving and your mind starts to wander, loop back to the original task in your mind. Reward yourself after completing the circuit with a short break and refocus.

Cleaning

Focus on one area at a time and move clockwise through the room, then the entire house. In each room, take out the trash first because it's a big, easy win. Next, remove everything from the counters. After those surfaces are clean, put everything in its place. Then you can move furniture and clean the floors. If you have trouble cleaning, take "before and after" photos for accountability and send them to an accountability buddy.

Laundry

Do laundry once a week, including bedsheets. Fold clothes while watching a show, listening to an audiobook or music playlist. You can use the runtime as a timer and it makes the work more enjoyable.

Meal planning

Make a stack of 5-10 recipe cards that hit all the bases for you and aren't too difficult. Use these recipes to create your grocery list. Besides the ingredients you'll need, add some quick, healthy snacks like nuts, fruit, and rice crackers.

Your grocery list needs to account for your household's needs in terms of quantity, taste preferences, and nutritional requirements. Focus on proteins and vegetables to build meals around. Involve your family and give them a choice by allowing them to select meals for the week and asking them to help brainstorm new recipes.

You can make a big batch of one recipe on the weekend and freeze it for quick meals or plan to make the same meal each weekday, like 'Taco Tuesday' and 'Spaghetti Wednesday'. These tactics save time and reduce daily decision fatigue.

Keep a shopping list taped to the inside of your pantry door and note what you need to buy more of. If the list is easily accessible, it will be easy to add to it and improve it. Keep a copy of your lists in your car and on your phone, so you can't leave them behind.

Shopping

- Keep copies of your shopping list in the car, in the kitchen, and on your phone.

- Keep reusable shopping bags in the car and by your launchpad so you always have some on hand.

- Stick to the perimeter of the store for healthier choices.

- Think about what you'll be eating based on what is in your cart.

- Check your cart before leaving.

Storage

- Organize your food by frequency of use.

- Always check what's in the back to prevent food from collecting dust or spoiling.

- Everything should have a special place so you can sort and find food quickly.

- Make a diagram or map of the kitchen organization scheme.

Cooking

1. Organize your ingredients

Wash your ingredients and place them on the counter in bowls. Also, get out any cookware you'll need.

2. Prep ingredients

This can be the most daunting step. Buy pre-cut veggies or bagged salad. Take a break after doing prep, so you don't get burned out.

3. Cook and combine

Use timers to prevent overcooking anything if you get distracted. Some people feel like they need to follow a recipe meticulously, but it helps to cultivate a sense of proper ingredient ratios. Learn what each ingredient and seasoning brings to the dish, add in small amounts, and taste often. If you leave food on the stove, leave the overhead light on too. That way, you will be less likely to forget about it.

4. Enjoy yourself

This is a creative process and there is no wrong answer.

Cooking shortcuts

- Bagged salad and pre-cut veggies
- Frozen or canned veggies
- Pasta and bread
- Breakfast for dinner
- Hard-boiled eggs
- Vegetable chopper

Cleanup

Clean the fridge and pantry regularly. Throw away spoiled foods and things you'll never eat.

Clean up as you go. It's easy to wash a few items as you wait for the water to boil, for instance. Don't fill the sink with large pots, cutting boards, and knives; it's much easier to quickly scrub those items before the food dries on and the sink is full. You'll be that much closer to chilling out after the meal. Reward yourself with other distractions only when the kitchen is clean.

7. Finances

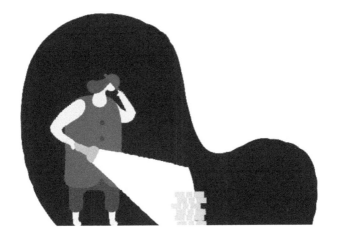

Finances are an area where it is important to have help. Banking apps, a savvy significant other, or a financial advisor can be crucial to getting your finances on track. I won't waste your time with advice on spending less money and making more money. You've heard it all before. The truth is, money can only come more easily to you when you are living as your best self. Do your best, work hard, and accept what you can't control.

- Keep a file for financial documents.

- Develop a budget and forecast your financial needs.

- Only keep small amounts of money on hand to prevent impulsive spending.

- Keep a wish list of things you'd like to buy.

8. Time

Judging the passage of time

Learn how long it takes you to do routine tasks at work and home. How long does it take to clean the kitchen? Do the laundry? Check your emails? We often misjudge the time spent on tasks due to a positive illusory bias, hyperfocus, and "now/not now" thinking. Misjudging time makes it very difficult to set accurate deadlines and is frustrating for everyone involved.

Set a timer for the next three times you perform these tasks. Alternatively, set a music playlist so you can judge the passage of time by how many songs have played since you started. Record these times in your treatment notebook or on a spreadsheet so you can become aware of how long things take and get ahead of time management.

One last thing

"One last thing before I go," often leads to rushing, stress, and mistakes. Everyone and everything in your way becomes a source of annoyance. Two alarms can help; a wrap-up warning and a second for 'hard end' time.

Time management

- Be prepared to overcome frustration. Show up for yourself.
- Be on time.
- Set alarms in different places.
- Set them for starting and stopping times.
- Avoid doing one last thing which can easily lead to never switching tasks.
- Make time external and visible with timers, calendars, reminders, and playlists.
- Schedule fun first.
- Schedule buffer time.
- Cut in half what you would normally set out to do.
- Schedule planning meetings with yourself.
- Divide your day into quadrants or thirds based on the number of tasks you can do that day.
- Don't get stuck planning.
- Write your current task on a big sheet of blank paper.
- See the big and little picture.
- Tell someone about your goals for accountability.

9. Home Treatment Plan

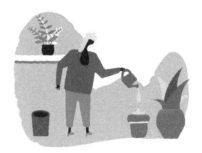

Choose a distraction to diminish or an area to improve in the home. You can change the stimuli to improve your behavioral patterns almost automatically. Focus on the benefits you will enjoy by making these changes.

- Distraction to diminish:
- Reason to address:
- Tactics:
- Area for improvement:
- Reason to improve:
- Tactics:

ADHD SOCIAL

Introduction

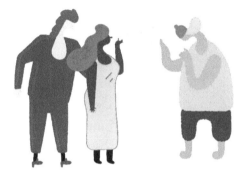

Social treatments build on the abilities enhanced by the previous two treatment types to improve your relationships with other people, yourself, and your projects. Stronger social skills will enable you to be more effective and get more joy out of life. Learn to manage conflicts, communicate more clearly, support others, and maintain strong relationships.

1. Communicating with Others

Your relationships could be the greatest source of happiness or unhappiness in life. How you communicate with your family and friends is a model for how you are in all of your relationships. We aspire to communicate clearly, honestly, and directly to minimize social anxiety and misunderstandings.

Some of the most important communications we have with others are non-verbal. Let's first examine how non-verbal cues influence the perception of your status.

Status

Your status has nothing to do with your value. Instead, it refers to how we interact with others. Do you carry yourself in a way that indicates you expect to be listened to? Or do you tend to defer to others and avoid responsibility? The former is high-status and the latter, low-status. So, are you generally a high-status or low-status person?

Indicators include your posture, the way you speak, move, and react; your general vibe. It is communicated in your bearing, how you treat others, and how you allow others to treat you. Your status is always changing and falls somewhere on a binary spectrum between high-status and low-status. Atypicals tend to exhibit low-status, are compliant, or hyper-reactive with erratic energy, speech, and movement.

Suggestions for communicating high-status:

- Make direct eye contact.
- Speak in complete sentences from your stomach.
- Breathe evenly and hold your head high.
- Adopt expansive postures and don't fidget.
- Don't telegraph your thoughts or feelings with your body language or tone.
- Don't telegraph your effort, even when a task is difficult for you.
- Pause and consider new information without telegraphing an impulsive reaction.

High status comes from making decisions and sticking to them with assuredness. Don't get defensive when you receive push-back. You don't need to be liked by others. Freedom from external acceptance is the ultimate expression of internal power.

Of course, everyone bounces between high and low-status, even in a single conversation. It doesn't matter where you gravitate on the status spectrum as long as you love yourself and protect your self-esteem like gold. It is gold.

Boundaries

Where is your yes and your no? If it's not a 'Hell yeah', then it's a 'No'.

Boundaries are clear definitions of how we expect to be treated. If you have a history of your boundaries being violated, they can be very difficult to perceive, and you might trample the boundaries of others without realizing it. Respect for boundaries is something to work on with a therapist.

Domino reactions

One of your symptoms triggers a reaction from another person, which causes you to react to their reaction. This is the formula for most habitual patterns of negative social interaction: symptom, response, response. It's persistent and automatic due to the involvement of rising emotions. This pattern can easily end in hopelessness and resentment. Learn to identify this pattern early by naming the steps, then plan for how you can defuse them.

Preventing domino reactions

- Monitor your feelings of anger and withdrawal.
- Keep respect for the other person and yourself.
- Use "I" statements rather than "you" statements. "I felt that…"
- Evaluate the facts of the situation and respond rationally, not emotionally.

- Use a panic word and take a break if it gets emotional.

- Be aware of your impulsivity and hypersensitivity.

- Breathe and let emotions pass. Imagine how a compassionate friend would talk to you about how you're feeling and why. What solutions could they offer?

- Control the controllable (your own actions) and let the rest go.

Addicted to bad feelings

Even bad feelings release brain chemicals and they can be just as addictive as the neurochemicals produced by positive behaviors. We learn to crave them on a set routine. Stronger feelings create more intense neurochemical releases, so we can get more of a rush by seeking stimulation from strong relationships. We might bait someone into bad feelings, just to get a fix. This is conflict as entertainment.

Bad stimulating behaviors include:

- Manufacturing a problem
- Being overly negative
- Blaming others and making excuses
- Demeaning and taking advantage to exercise power

Bottom line it

Avoid rambling by starting with your point. State things succinctly and clearly. It might be blunt, but that's better than wasting time vaguely circling an issue. Inability to state what you want can be related to discomfort with confrontation. That is something to talk about with a therapist.

2. Friends

Focus on the other person with your whole body. The best listening happens when we look at the person who is talking. We often look around while listening and become sidetracked by our own thoughts. This type of body language is not conducive to building a strong friendship. If you lose focus, ask them to repeat themselves.

Say yes, say no

Atypicals tend to be very agreeable and want to say yes. This behavior leads to a long to-do list, which can get overwhelming quickly. Protect your time and remember that whenever you say yes to something, you are saying no to every other possibility. Otherwise, you will begin to break obligations and be seen as an unreliable friend.

Digital agenda

Tell your friends about your efforts to limit distraction, especially as it pertains to communication on social media and other persistent distractions.

Social tips

- Know yourself and your interests.
- Make soft commitments rather than an unqualified "yes."
- Stay aware of your schedule.
- Note the small things, like birthdays.
- Get feedback.
- Don't get trapped somewhere you don't want to be. Make an exit plan.
- Be direct and upfront.
- Don't take things personally.
- Interested is interesting.
- Do nice things for important people in your life.
- Develop interests and passions.
- Passion comes from action, not the other way around.

3. Significant Other

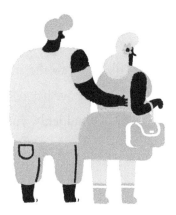

Courtship is exhilarating and atypicals tend to be good at creative acts of romance. Long-term relationships, however, present challenges that can be difficult to overcome because emotional stress makes treatment more difficult.

Hyperfocus shock

Atypicals tend to be alluring partners in the beginning stages of a relationship. You have lots of energy, creative spirit and are hyperfocused on your partner. After the honeymoon phase, however, your partner may be blindsided by the sudden change when your hyperfocus shifts. This change can make them feel confused and neglected. Are you the same person they fell in love with? Has something changed about the relationship? No, your brain has simply switched to hyperfocus on something else. It will take your partner some time to adjust.

Positive illusory bias

Positive illusory bias sets atypicals up to be blindsided by a failing relationship. We are oblivious to the strain caused by our inconsistency, neglect, and impulsive behavior. We believe that everything is going well, then, suddenly, your partner is upset with you.

- You: "What do you mean you're leaving me? I thought everything was great."
- Your partner: "Of course you think it's great! I do everything and get nothing from you!"

Your symptoms can make it difficult to manage certain tasks. Focus on our physiological treatments and slowly add responsibilities that you can handle. Your partner can help you as you strengthen these areas, but be sure to compensate in other areas and continue to improve. You don't want to slide into a parent-child dynamic with your partner. Set boundaries to diminish the parent-child relationship.

Parent-child dynamic

When your partner feels that they are shouldering an unfair amount of the responsibility in a relationship, they may begin to view you as a child. The parent-child dynamic quickly sours any romantic feelings and leads to resentment. Set clear boundaries and show that you are managing your responsibilities with actions.

Common relationship problems for atypicals

- Think only of yourself
- Forgetful of important dates and obligations
- Taking advantage of your partner for reminders and stability
- Consistently undependable, breaking promises
- Never finishes projects
- Can't keep a job
- Doesn't express interest in partner's projects
- Neglects romantic responsibilities
- Promises to do better but doesn't follow through
- Misunderstands the feelings and intentions of others
- Dishonest behavior
- Never on time

Fighting

Fights are good, and healthy anger is desirable. They communicate our needs. Don't suppress anger or shy away from conflict. It is rage and resentment which are toxic. Also, the number or the severity of your fights are unimportant; it's important how and why you make up.

Relationships are difficult for everyone. You can only control your own happiness and growth, so don't suffer trying to make someone else be happy.

Often, your significant other getting angry with you boils down to a misunderstood expectation of you. Identify the expectation and compare it to the reality so you can find solutions without resorting to rage or shame.

Three stages

In order to establish realistic expectations, it can be useful to think of your treatment progress in three stages.

1. Denial of symptoms

2. Acceptance and action to diminish symptoms

3. Effectively managed symptoms

Strive for stage three, but accept that, for most symptoms, you will always be at stage two and that's OK. As long as you can get past stage one, progress is possible.

Learning conversations

The person who is feeling upset starts the conversation with an 'I' statement and explains the issue in two or three brief sentences. "I need" and "I feel" instead of "you always" or "you never." Then, their partner demonstrates that they understand the issue by explaining it in their own words. This should continue until both partners feel that the issue is understood. When the listener gets it right, they switch roles. Maintain respect and dignity, avoid toxicity.

Safe word

Set a verbal cue that either partner can use when you feel yourself becoming emotionally flooded and argumentative. Past this point, nothing productive can actually occur, so it's best just to take a break and come back when progress is possible.

Partner check-ins

Plan to check in once a week to talk about progress and goals. It will help you stay coordinated, voice concerns, and feel like a team.

Also, protect mealtimes so there is always a pleasant reason to gather, enjoy each other's company, and address issues.

Apologizing

Do not qualify your apology. Take responsibility. Address feelings of resentment, symptoms, and the issues they caused for others. Be there for your partner with your time and attention. How can you do that best? Remember, it is not about how you think things are. It is about how they feel. How can you make your partner feel supported and special?

Kids

There is a good chance your children inherited your ADHD just as you almost certainly did from your parents. Be a role model. Don't hide the effort you put into managing your household.

Regardless of whether your children are atypical, you need to make them feel important to you. If you are late picking them up from school, apologize and make a plan so it doesn't happen again. Be honest without complaint or excuse. That sort of behavior makes people feel insecure, which is counter to your responsibilities as a parent.

Extended Family

Anyone outside of you and your direct dependents is a secondary priority. They will need to take care of themselves until you are strong enough to manage more responsibility. Unless they are part of your treatment team, your extended family can be a distraction or even an obstacle. Take responsibility for these relationships; be firm and say what you need.

4. Social Treatment Plan

Reflect on the interpersonal aspect of your life. Choose an area that you could strengthen, whether that's a specific relationship or a symptom that affects your social interactions more broadly. Ask yourself why you want to improve this area. How could you do it? Come up with several options and set a time on your calendar to follow through with action.

- Target symptom:
- Reason to improve:
- Tactics:

ADHD WORK
& SCHOOL

Introduction

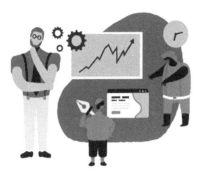

Your work situation can be broken into three components; the tasks involved, the environment, and the other people like your boss/teacher, coworkers, and clients. Our workplaces can be the most unforgiving in terms of treatments available and the ability to control stress. In each area, control the controllable, implement a structure that works for you, and don't settle for misery. Use your strengths to overcome weaknesses.

Most treatments are applicable to both work and school, but specific tips for each are provided in the final chapters of this section.

1. Obstacles

The same symptoms that make life difficult for atypicals affect our workplace and school situation. A brief recap of stand-out issues would include:

- Impulsivity
- Procrastination
- Poor executive function
- Poor communication
- Poor time perception
- Poor attention to details
- Trouble switching between tasks

In addition to those listed above, a few other symptoms should be noted in the workplace context.

Sapience

The ability to figure out how to behave without being told is called sapience. Atypicals are often oblivious to the unwritten rules of a setting. Sapience governs your ability to act with appropriate judgment. Observe your coworkers and talk to an ally about unwritten office rules for clarification.

Harassment

Don't tolerate harassment. Light joking and teasing are OK as long as everyone is OK with it. Atypicals often struggle with addressing conflict, but this is an opportunity to be direct. Describe the problematic behavior and ask that it stop. Record each instance of harassment and include dates. If the harassment continues, bring the record to a superior. Having the specific dates and exact quotations that offended you will help you manage the emotional stress.

Overwork

Don't suffer in silence. Set limits for what you can accomplish and communicate those boundaries. Ask for accommodations and focus on what you can do, not what you can't. This conversation can be difficult but is better than burning out from stress or letting people down when you can't meet unrealistic expectations.

Impulsivity

Response inhibition is our ability to suppress immediate reactions and choose between several options, your mental brakes. Take it slow and follow through on your original intention first. Controlling impulsivity generally improves with age.

Wandering communication

Bottom-line it. State your point clearly first, so you don't talk in circles.

Write down your thoughts before speaking face-to-face. Have an ally review your thought process before big decisions.

Overcommitment

Only do what you want to do. It's OK to think about it, consult your schedule, or say no.

- "Let me think about it and get back to you."
- "I wish I could help, but I can't."
- "I can't do that, but I could…"
- "No."

Impatience and unrealistic expectations

Get a realistic perspective on the amount of work it takes to succeed at your goal. Ask others how long their days are or how many hours they work or study for an exam. Otherwise, you may get frustrated for no good reason.

Performance Anxiety

A history of not doing well can become a self-fulfilling prophecy and you can become anxious just thinking about taking a test or starting a task. The anxiety itself becomes the focus.

Overcoming performance anxiety

- Identify the thoughts causing you anxiety and try to modify them.

- Accept the anxiety, the uncontrollable, and your limitations.

- Work on your mental attitude and put this challenge in perspective. It is of small significance in the greater context of your life. It is not a measure of who you are.

- Start preparing well in advance.

- Learn different strategies to attack your obstacles.

- Seek accommodations if time constraints or other factors are distracting.

- Arrive early; early is on time.

- Grab low-hanging fruit first to build confidence.

Other common work/study problems

- Poor concentration
- Poor time management
- Difficulty integrating information
- Difficulty prioritizing and selecting main ideas
- Unclear directions
- Lack of motivation

Focused distraction

Manual drivers with ADHD are safer because they are constantly being reminded to maintain focus by operating the car. Preoccupy your restless mind with a focused form of distraction like taking notes, gripping a stress ball, or taking a walk. A focused distraction will keep you sharp and can make you appear more engaged.

2. Coworkers, Clients & Workspace

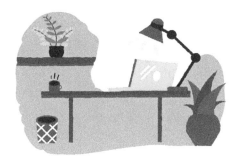

Coworkers & Clients

Most people like atypicals at first because of our natural charismatic appeal. Then they get let down again and again until it is too much, and the relationship ends. Remember, you are not a bad person. You have problematic behaviors; the behavior is bad. You can change the behavior. Be consistent, communicate directly, and ask for clarification.

Workspace

You will have less control over your environment at work than at home. Nevertheless, you should be able to run a similar analysis of distractions and available treatments to make improvements.

3. Project Planning

Your ideas are not a plan until they are written down in concrete terms. Don't avoid taking the time that planning demands. It is part of the process that we often rush through in a panic of last minute haste. If planning is difficult, it will require additional time and effort.

Consider the suggestions below as you take the time to write the steps of each of your plans on their corresponding calendar events:

- Understand the objective.

- Set a goal and determine what milestones are to achieve it.

- Plan backward to now.

- Prioritize.

- Set deadlines for milestones and add them to the calendar.

- Make an event for each milestone on its respective deadline.

- Break the milestones into tasks.

- Add task lists to each milestone calendar event.

- Create a to-do list for your next milestone.

- Choose a reasonable number of daily tasks.

- Tasks should be refined to the smallest, simplest actions.

- Gather materials and execute the actions.

- Time yourself, leave transition time, record your results on the calendar.

- Reward yourself.

- Evaluate progress and adjust deadlines.

- Communicate progress to other team members.

Barriers to organization

- Always rushing

- Impulsively placing things anywhere

- Poor classification and categorization of items

- Constantly overcommitting

- Leaving no time to plan or organize

- Distractibility

- Feeling overwhelmed by setbacks

- Procrastination and indecisiveness

- "Shoot, then aim" approach to problem-solving

- Not collecting necessary information

- Not considering all possible solutions
- Lacking the patience to develop a plan
- Struggling to muster attention
- Impulsively going with the first thing that comes to mind

4. Communication

Workplace interactions require additional considerations beyond normal social interaction. Most jobs demand that you communicate precisely, execute tasks reliably, and observe special rules of conduct. The following tips will help smooth workplace communication.

Personal issues

Growing up, you may have been criticized or rejected for reasons you didn't understand. You may have particular triggers and sensitive areas that cause you to become upset or angry quickly. This will be confusing to the people you are with now.

It is inappropriate to discuss these personal issues with most people who aren't close friends. Try to leave your past behind you. Therapy helps with this.

Small talk

Learn the importance of small talk. It greases the skids of social interaction. It is the work of mining social currency and finding connections with people, which can turn into real benefits. Know when a conversation is ending. Don't drag out goodbyes.

FORDs

This is an acronym for Family, Occupation, Recreation, and Dreams. These are four relatively safe topics of conversation that are relatable and get people to talk about themselves. Build multiple FORDs with someone and small talk will be much easier. Try to remember some details because the small stuff counts with people when you are trying to show them that you care.

Remembering names

Create a system to remember people's names. If you forget, let them know you have trouble with names and ask them to remind you. Most people are OK with this. It's better than expecting the other person to correct you.

Relationship assuredness

Be assertive about what you need. Don't be passive. Create interactions with people that have energy in them. Even if you make someone mad, you are in a relationship with them. They wouldn't be mad if they didn't care about the relationship in some way. They would just walk away.

More communication tips

- You are communicating constantly, even by avoiding communication.

- Be aware of your language. Be aware of your tone and volume. Match the other person's level of emotion and personal disclosure.

- Avoid assumptions. No one can read minds. Clarify with questions.

- Repeat what someone has said in your own words, paraphrase.

- Be patient. Take regular pauses in conversation. Become comfortable with silence.

- Respect boundaries. Do not intrude on others' personal space.

- Wait to make major decisions.

- See the good in others.

- Stand firm when things go wrong.

- Surround yourself with positive people.

- Let people know when you are switching topics so your thoughts are easier to follow.

- Acknowledge when you interrupt and apologize. Take notes so that you don't get anxious about forgetting your idea.

- Speak in short sentences that communicate clearly, as if you were being interviewed on TV. Listen more than you talk.

- Writing your thoughts down solidifies them and makes them easier to express. Set a mutual agenda for the conversation at the outset.

- Think before you speak: Is it true? Is it important? Is it relevant to what is being said?

- Keep the other person's purpose in mind.

- Show interest with your body language. Don't multitask while talking.

- Express confidence and positivity.

- Ask rather than tell.

- Choose the right place, time and style of conversation setting. Minimize competing stimuli. If you feel restless, suggest a walk and talk.

- Pause if you feel emotional.

- Be clear about follow-up.

- Be gracious, speak diplomatically.

- In confrontations, maintain respect and dignity, avoid toxicity, and take responsibility.

5. Pay Attention

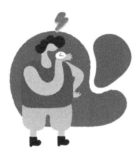

Although most of these tips have been covered, the following is a review of the most important tips for communicating that you are engaged in workplace conversations.

- Listen with your body.
- Choose the right environment.
- Use a focused distraction like note taking.
- Set parameters for the duration and topics to be covered.

Reflect on recent conversations

Can you repeat specifics about the conversation? What did they ask you to do? What details about time, dates, and plans do you remember? Did you listen as much as you talked? Did you focus? Did you drift? Did you learn something about the other person you didn't know before? Did this conversation deepen the relationship or positively move toward some other positive objective?

Repeat it in your own words, write it down, or ask for clarification in a follow-up email.

Commit to change

Do you want to change anything about your communication? Write down specifics about what you want to accomplish. Prioritize these goals and review them regularly. Reflection is the basis of a personality makeover. You are becoming a new person. Not changing, but revealing your best self that was present all along.

6. Follow Through

Atypicals are great at ideas, but struggle with execution. The actions required to turn ideas into reality are just as important as the ideas themselves. Keep the following tips in mind to maintain conscious effort and follow through.

- Don't overcommit.
- Consider your other obligations before you make a promise.
- Ask yourself if you have the skills and information necessary.
- Check your current obligations before a meeting and don't volunteer for something before doing so.
- Don't do things just to be nice.
- Once you commit, write down specifically what needs to be done and when.
- Make yourself a timeline.

- Let others know quickly if you probably won't be able to deliver on time.

- Don't volunteer the services of someone else without checking first.

- Let people know if you won't have time to do something, or negotiate a way to reduce your other responsibilities so that you do have time.

- Allow yourself some transition time to pause and review your progress before starting a new activity.

7. Finding the Right Path

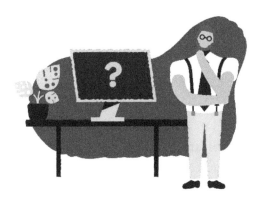

When you understand your values, strengths, and weak points, it becomes possible to consider your ideal work. What is your ideal work? What is your ideal workplace? What would it take to make a change in that direction?

You may be reluctant to leave your current job for one that is better suited, but rest assured that, once you find something you are excited about, you will love working at it. Your perception of work may be skewed from spending time at a job you hate because it is a grind and a struggle to keep up with expectations that don't suit you.

Your passion and excitement will return when you find the right fit. To find the right fit, think of the times in your life when you've felt "in the zone," when time flew by. What were you doing when you liked yourself best? Can you translate that activity into a career? Professional career counselors can help fine-tune this discovery process as well.

Even if you are satisfied in your current position or can't leave it, consider what improvements could be made. Change begins the moment we make our desires known. It won't be perfect, but it can be better. Progress, not perfection.

Finding a good match for your strengths

Find your purpose, your sweet spot. Consider your strengths and what careers are a match for those strengths. You are more likely to succeed in a career that plays to your strengths. Understand your personality and learning style. Write a list of unique traits. They might be ADHD-related but aren't disorders or deficits. Find an area of interest suited to you. What activities make time seem to go quickly and put you in the "flow state?"

Characteristics of jobs suited to atypicals

- Fast pace with varied tasks each day
- You can move around or travel during the day
- Intellectually stimulating or challenging

- There are firm due dates for projects
- You receive frequent feedback and expectations are clear
- The schedule is flexible
- There is immediate reinforcement for a job well done

Entrepreneurs

This could be a dream or a nightmare. You set the agenda, but you are solely responsible. Atypicals tend to be great idea people because they think differently and synthesize ideas with ease. Most businesses succeed because of a great team of people supporting the vision, so make sure you develop strong relationships, leadership qualities, and partner with people who have complementary skills.

8. Accommodations

Accommodations are compromises that are agreed upon to help you succeed. They don't make things easier; they remove some stress and give you time to improve. Accommodations are handled at an administrative level. Without formal accommodations, some supervisors will help you out; others won't. With accommodations, everyone must.

I want to do a great job, but when coworkers constantly interrupt me, I get derailed. Would it be OK to work on this project in a different room?

Disclosing your condition

Reserve your privacy at work until you've thought through the consequences of identifying yourself as someone in need of accommodations. Schools are usually very accommodating. Friends should bring out your best and compensate for your weaknesses. Be your own best friend.

Learn to advocate for yourself and speak clearly and unemotion-
ally about how ADHD affects your performance. Establish clear
expectations in your relationships and boundaries on how you
want to be treated. Agree to call a timeout if emotions run hot.

Steps for requesting accommodations

1. Make an appointment with your teacher or
   supervisor to discuss your condition.

2. Assemble persuasive reasons for accommodations based on your shared goals.

3. Confirm your needs by stating what you'd like
   to accomplish.

4. Clarify what compromise you are asking for
   and justify your needs.

5. Reach an agreement and record the details by
   following up by email. Forward it to anyone
   who might need to be in the loop.

The law

The ADA (Americans with Disabilities Act) lists ADHD as a
disability. You are legally eligible for accommodations. They
aren't specific but could include flextime, visual cues, organization systems, treatment subsidies.

At this time, most experts recommend not disclosing your condition because many employers will use this information against
you. It is uncommon for an employer to provide accommodations, and few win employment discrimination lawsuits. Your
best bet is to seek informal accommodations.

9. School Tips

Our responsibilities at work and school can be similar in terms of scrutiny from others, but the freedom we are granted and the way we define success are different. There are several tips that apply specifically to choosing an area of interest, studying, and completing academic tasks like tests and homework.

Consider the following tips to improve your outcomes at school:

- Get the books you need and read them.
- Read the syllabus.
- Go to every class, sit in the front, take notes, ask questions, engage.
- Write assignments in your planner.
- Make a study schedule for tests.
- Do the homework and readings, be prepared.
- You can't study and party.
- Talk to the instructors, think of questions to expand your knowledge and areas of interest.

- Don't procrastinate.
- Take breaks.
- Pick a good place and time to study.
- Start with the hard stuff.
- Make sure you understand the assignment.
- Sit in a comfortable chair.
- Work with others when appropriate.
- No one is making you gain knowledge; you get to.
- Reflect on what you are learning and make a conscious effort to recall the information.

10. Workplace Tips

The workplace is a source of special stress. Our responsibilities and systems of accountability are often more rigidly defined than in our personal lives. Instead of dreading this reality, use it to your advantage. Clarity is one of the most important aspects of overcoming procrastination and moving forward.

Below are more tips that will benefit you in any work environment:

- Take frequent short breaks.

- Replace fluorescents, which can cause a distracting buzz.

- Allow extra time for meetings and events, so you don't overbook yourself.

- Ask for an office free from distractions.

- Avoid cubicles which often have inherent and unavoidable distractions.

- Keep your hands busy by taking notes during meetings as an intentional distraction.

- Insist on clear deadlines and clarify what is expected of you; make a paper trail.

- Break everything into smaller chunks.

- Schedule challenging work for when you are sharpest.

- Buddy up with a coworker for accountability.

- Get to work 15 minutes early to prepare for the day; early is on time.

- Ask for flexibility so you can alter your work-day's start and end times.

- Use time management apps and alarms.

- Employ a color-coded organization system.

- Schedule meetings with your boss to make sure you're on track.

- Spell check everything twice.

- Carry a small notebook for popcorn thoughts and your daily checklist.

- Set time limits for email and other tasks that could distract you.

- Take time at the end of the day to organize and prepare for tomorrow.

- Separate the setup from the task.

- Use rewards as good stress. If a friend asks you to go out, say you have to work for three solid hours, or you must cancel. The stress of wanting something can sometimes switch on your hyperfocus.

- Set a realistic deadline and an aspirational deadline.

- Make actions concrete by making SMART goals.

- Create safe, high stakes. Don't take a laptop charger with you to the coffee shop and let the battery draining motivate you.

- Understand what prevents you from following through and work around it.

11. Work & School Action Plan

Work and academic settings provide abundant opportunities for feedback. Use this feedback to target specific weaknesses and choose treatment tactics to improve them.

- Target symptom:
- Reason to improve:
- Tactics:

CONCLUSION

Awareness, Intention & Action

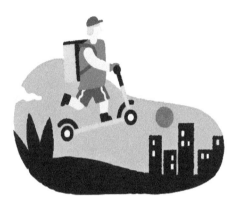

Ultimately, three ideals will determine your treatment outcomes: awareness, intention, and action. If you find yourself struggling, start with the problem and work backward, considering the situation through each of these lenses. Do I understand the situation? Do I know what I want? What must I do to get it?

Improving these cornerstones is the work of a lifetime and is not a challenge exclusive to atypicals. Everyone needs to strengthen these areas, and the work is never done. Let's review them in detail one more time.

Awareness

1. *Observe*

Observe the situation and identify how and why you'd like it to change. Be aware of emotions, behaviors and habits.

2. *Understand & Accept*

Accept your condition and its challenges. Admit that many struggles are a result of your condition and separate yourself from your behaviors. Establish some emotional distance between who you are as a person and the symptoms of your condition.

Intention

1. *Choose a target*

Choose one issue to start working on. Look at your symptoms and decide what's causing you the most trouble. Have one small goal. Narrow in on the negative patterns and behaviors that prevent you from attaining your goal so you can develop countermeasures to overcome them.

2. *Decide on an action and gather your tools*

"My goal is to modify (problematic behavior) by doing (treatment) so that I can change the behavior to (adaptive behavior)."

3. *Plan*

Focus on your strengths when making your plan. Imagine you are a general with a special mission that was specifically drafted for you based on your strengths.

"I see that this person is good at X. Here is how the plan uses those strengths."

Action

1. Execute the plan

Work and follow the plan without second-guessing. It's not quick and easy. Refuse to give up. Reject the idea when you confront it. Push against it to propel yourself forward. Write yourself a letter to be opened three weeks from now, which lists your most likely obstacles and feelings. Remind yourself why you are moving forward. Repeat your mantra. Get an accountability partner.

2. Evaluate

Evaluate your progress regularly. Slow down. What is working? Why is it working? How can I track my progress? If something isn't working, what about it isn't? What can I do about that? When will I do it? What is my commitment level? How can I remember my commitment? Give your strategy enough time to work and take the time to evaluate your plan. Be prepared for frustration.

If you get sidetracked, ask:

- Am I repeating an old pattern?
- Do I want to quit from boredom?
- Is wanting to quit part of the old pattern?
- Am I separating the action from myself?

ERIC ANDERSON

- How can I make the plan more enticing so that I will follow through?
- How does my plan support my mission statements?

3. *Repeat*

Repeat the process and don't regress. Don't stop. That's the hardest and most important part. Keep stomping through failures toward new successes. Use what's working in one aspect of your life and apply it to other areas. Be compassionate and reward yourself.

Afterword

Congratulations, you have ADHD and you are on the path to treatment. Big steps. ADHD is a hopeful diagnosis because it demonstrates your understanding and willingness to improve your quality of life.

ADHD is not a gift, a curse, or an excuse. It is an explanation and it comes with difficulties. It is an understanding of the way your brain operates. Understanding your behavior puts formerly impossible obstacles into an approachable context. It opens the door to change. Your problems are not who you are; they are a group of treatable symptoms.

There's no such thing as a fresh start. You need your past. Own it, or it will own you. From now on, you have the power to fundamentally alter how you see yourself and interact with the world. Every one of your relationships will improve by accepting this power. There are no clean slates, only redemption through improvement.

ADHD does not limit your potential. It enhances certain potentials. It differentiates you. It allows you to forgive the mistakes of your past self and build a future that is tailored to your personal needs.

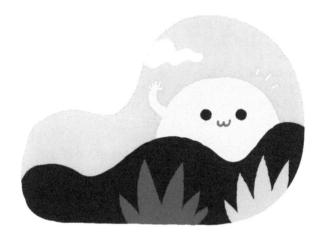

Wherever you go, there you are.

INDEX

A

Accommodations 48, 221, 223, 240, 241
Advocate for yourself 241
Americans with Disabilities Act 241
Anger 33, 35, 46, 47, 129, 171, 206, 214
ANTs 130, 131, 134, 172
Aristotle 115
Attention to details 21, 220
Atypicals 22, 23, 32, 34, 38, 42, 48, 49, 70, 79, 93, 96, 104, 110, 129, 135,
    138, 147, 149, 153, 158, 166, 169, 170, 205, 209, 211, 212, 213,
    220, 221, 225, 235, 238, 239, 249
Aurelius, Marcus 119
Awareness 27, 38, 39, 58, 59, 96, 134, 139, 143, 155, 249, 250

B

Blame 27, 34, 126, 127
Bottom line it 208
Buddy up 245

C

Calendar 66, 68, 69, 70, 71, 72, 73, 75, 78, 138, 165, 217, 226, 227
Cleaning 33, 185, 192
Clutter 98, 99, 182, 184, 185, 186, 187
    Divide the space 185
    Magic Bin 187
    Spot Cleaning 185
    Your Papers 186
Cognitive distortions 130
Communication 111, 209, 220, 222, 229, 230, 234
Courtship 211

Creativity myths 170
Crossroads Moments 66
Crushing ANTs 134

D

Daily checklist 68, 74, 79, 245
Denial 26, 46, 214
Diet 110, 111, 112, 117
Divergent thinkers 169
Divorce 20
Domino reactions 206

E

Emotional outburst therapy 142
Encoding and accessing learned information 16
Entrepreneurs 239
Environment 38, 39, 53, 57, 83, 85, 98, 99, 100, 134, 154, 160, 177, 178,
        180, 191, 219, 225, 233, 244
Evening check-in 69, 138, 156
Examine your outlook 140
Example mantras 145
Exercise 67, 77, 85, 91, 102, 105, 107, 108, 109, 114, 115, 117, 142, 154,
        168, 175, 207

F

Failure 16, 41, 51, 59, 60, 127, 128, 132, 133, 135, 136, 137, 152, 173
Feng Shui 100
Finances 178, 186, 197
Focused distraction 224, 233
FORDs 230
Friends 36, 39, 49, 55, 57, 64, 127, 144, 204, 209, 229, 240
Fun menu 164

G

Gamify tasks 165
Goal-setting 71
Good sleep 103

H

Hanger Trick 167
Hereditary condition 30, 37, 48
Hyperactivity 31, 33
Hyperfocus 31, 32, 34, 49, 85, 169, 185, 192, 199, 211, 212, 246

I

Ideal environment 98, 100
Impaired Executive Function 31, 32, 59
Impulsivity 21, 86, 142, 184, 207, 220, 221
Inattentiveness 18, 35
Inner castle 141
Inner child 121, 141
Inner guardian 141, 142
Insecurity 36, 40, 41
Insurance 45, 178
Intentional distractions 102

K

Kids 216

L

Labeling 133
Laziness 40
Long-term memory 149
Losing things 189, 190

M

Magnification or minimization 132
Maladaptive behaviors 16, 135
Managing emotional responses 16
Meal planning 193
Medication 25, 26, 27, 42, 49, 93, 94, 95, 96, 105, 111, 117
    Vacations 94
Method of Loci 149
Momentum 50, 156, 163

Monitoring and guiding your actions 16
Motivation 72, 153, 163, 223
Myths 18, 19, 170

N

Negative lens 134
Neuroatypical 22
Novel association 149, 189

O

Obstacles 38, 39, 40, 46, 53, 58, 60, 72, 93, 105, 120, 123, 125, 130, 135, 220, 223, 251, 252
Oppositional Defiant Disorder 31, 34
Organization 182, 183, 194, 227, 241, 245
    Barriers 227
    Benefits 182
Organizing 15, 32, 98, 185, 186
Outsource encouragement 151
Overcommitment 222
Overgeneralizing 131

P

Palette cleanser 155
Parent-child dynamic 212, 213
Pause, breathe, and accept 16
Perfectionism 39, 59, 137
Performance anxiety 222, 223
Personal Style 166
Perspective and choice 142
Physiological state 92
Plan in reverse 161
Planning 34, 100, 160, 161, 200, 226
Pomodoro Technique 79
Popcorn thoughts 78, 138, 245
Positive illusory bias 59, 199, 212
Presence 166, 167

Prioritizing tasks 156
Procrastination 36, 39, 59, 135, 136, 184, 220, 227, 244
    Distracted 136, 189, 190
    Forgetfulness 20, 136
    Ineffective prioritizing 136
    Overwhelmed 137
Progress 46, 54, 64, 68, 69, 70, 76, 78, 152, 163, 192, 214, 215, 227, 236, 238, 251
Project Planning 226

R

Reflection 78, 107, 137, 139, 177, 234
Regret and grief 46
Regulating self-control 15
Rejection Sensitive Dysphoria 31, 34
Relaxation 72, 73, 121, 165, 173
Relaxation and transition time 72
Reprogramming your habits 120
Routines 49, 51, 54, 65, 66, 67, 68, 77, 140, 150, 180

S

Sapience 220
School 32, 44, 64, 216, 219, 220, 242, 247
Self-blame 126
Self-defeating ideas 125
Self-diagnosis 43, 44
Self-esteem 24, 36, 107, 126, 127, 140, 166, 170, 205
Self-fulfilling prophecy 132, 222
Self-Medication 96, 97
Self-pity 127
Self-preservation 40
Self-shaming 132, 152
Sensory visualization 148, 186
Shifting focus 15
Shopping 81, 193, 194
Sidetracked 161, 209, 251
Soundscape 101
Stick to the plan 156

Stimulants 93, 94
Stop, breathe, and accept 28
Stress 33, 35, 41, 72, 73, 92, 94, 103, 110, 117, 120, 125, 136, 150, 161,
          162, 177, 184, 189, 199, 211, 219, 221, 224, 240, 244, 245
Suicide 20
Symptoms 16, 17, 18, 20, 22, 24, 25, 26, 30, 31, 35, 37, 39, 40, 44, 47, 49,
          59, 63, 91, 94, 95, 126, 127, 128, 169, 172, 206, 212, 214, 215, 220,
          250, 252

T

Task circuits 191
Time management 199, 200, 223, 245
Train station 115
Triggers 39, 83, 85, 86, 120, 124, 174, 180, 206, 229
Tzu, Lao 13

U

Understand & Accept 250
Urgency 41, 75, 79, 156, 186

V

Visual cues 66, 83, 180, 241

W

Wandering communication 222
Workspace 225

CPSIA information can be obtained
at www.ICGtesting.com
Printed in the USA
LVHW081655200223
739943LV00020B/824/J